MUSCLEMAG INTERNATIONAL'S

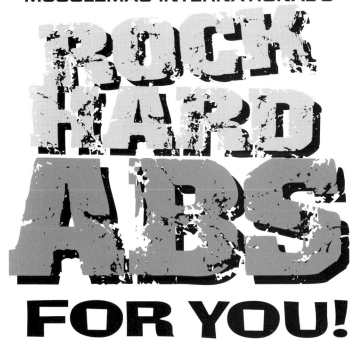

ROCK HARD ABS

FOR YOU!

Shape Up That Waistline

By Robert Kennedy & Dwayne Hines II

Rock Hard Abs For You! Shape Up That Waistline

Published by MuscleMag International
6465 Airport Road
Mississauga, ON
Canada L4V 1E4

Designed by Jackie Kydyk
Copy edited by Nancy LePatourel

10 9 8 7 6 5 4 3 2 1 Pbk

Canadian Cataloguing in Publication Data

Kennedy, Robert, 1938-
    Musclemag international's Rock hard abs for you! : shape up that waistline

ISBN 1-55210-017-0

    1. Abdominal exercises. I. Hines, Dwayne, 1961-
II. Title. III. Title: Rock hard abs for you.

RA781.6.K44 2000   646.7'5   C00-900211-1

Distributed in Canada by
CANBOOK Distribution Services
1220 Nicholson Road
Newmarket, ON
L3Y 7V1
800-399-6858

Distributed in the States by
BookWorld Services
1933 Whitfield Park Loop
Sarasota, FL 34243
800-444-2524

Printed in Canada

WARNING
This book is not intended as medical advice, nor is it offered for use in the diagnosis of any health condition or as a substitute for medical treatment and/or counsel. Its purpose is to explore advanced topics on sports nutrition and exercise. All data are for information only. Use of any of the programs within this book is at the sole risk and choice of the reader.

Table of Contents

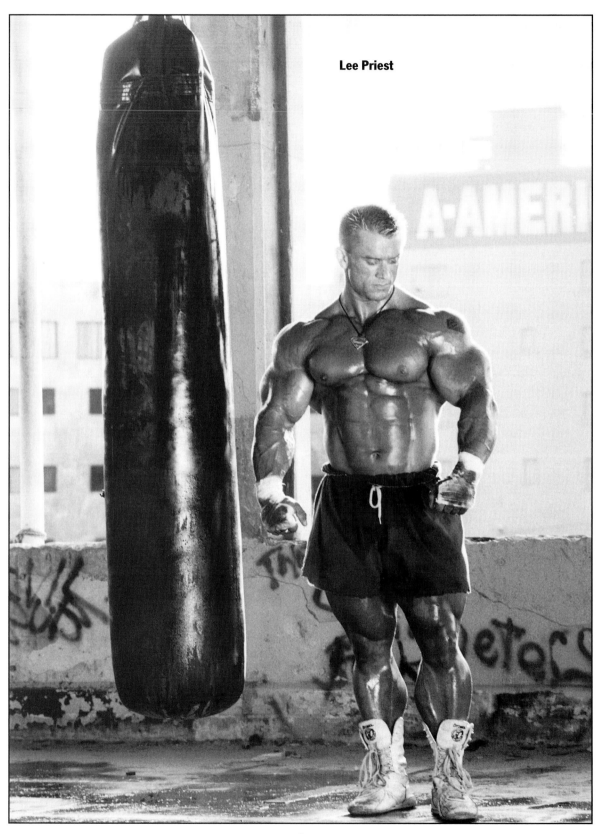

Lee Priest

Introduction

A well-sculpted stomach is the centerpiece of the physique. But just having a smaller stomach is no guarantee that your middle will look great. Many people have a mid-section that is not all that large, but is still non-descript because it lacks shape.

Slim and Shapely

A stomach that looks super is a stomach that is both slim and shapely, combining slender lines with sensuous curvature. The entire area must carry very little fat. This combination of slimness and shape is dynamite for the appearance.

> ### A super looking stomach combines slender lines with sensuous curvature.

Without a slender and shapely stomach, the overall body shape takes on one of two configurations. Either the stomach region "breaks even," which gives the body a non-descript average appearance, or it loses ground and gets too large, giving the body a rounded look in the middle. Although the first state is obviously better than the second, neither of these less than top conditions is something that you want.

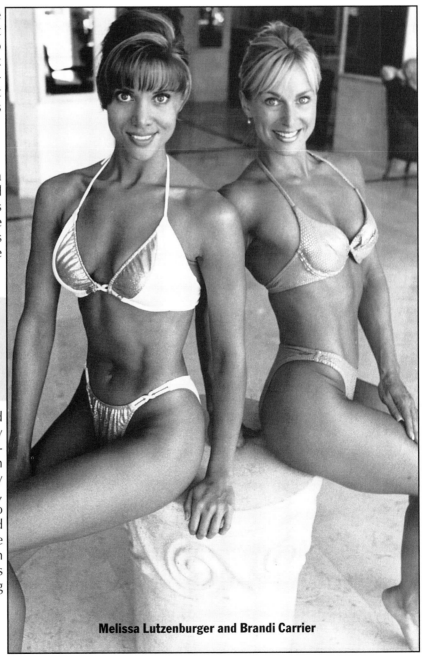

Melissa Lutzenburger and Brandi Carrier

The Fashionable Physique

A slim and shapely stomach looks good in clothing as well as in a swimsuit. In fact, one of the best things you can do to improve your fashion appearance is to reshape your stomach. This will positively change the way your clothes fit. Most people don't appear to realize the tremendous boost that a sharp looking physique gives their fashion appearance – and the condition of the waist is central to this appearance upgrade.

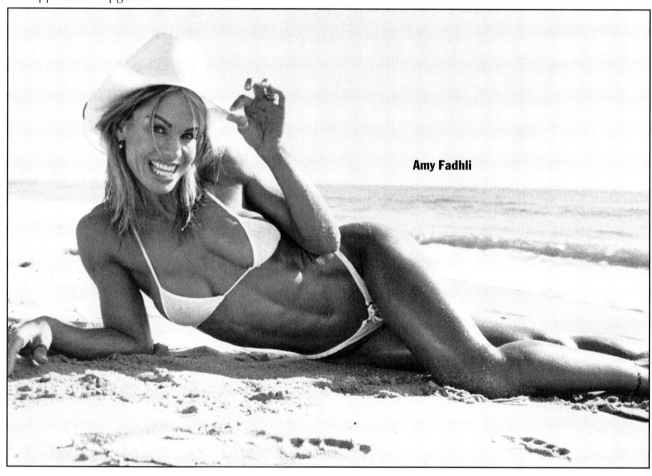

Amy Fadhli

A Healthy Body

In addition to the cosmetic enhancement that a slender and shapely stomach gives the body, there is also a corresponding health benefit. A general rule of thumb is that the more trim your waistline, the better your overall health condition. Of course this is not always the case, but it is a good general rule.

Researchers at the Harvard Medical School point out that it is not just excess weight, but an excessive waist that increases a woman's risk of adult-onset diabetes. Data compiled from over 42,000 women revealed that, compared with a 28-inch waistline, the risk for diabetes was two and a half times higher for a 30- to 31-inch waist; four times as high for a 32- to 33-inch waist; roughly four and a half times higher for a 34- to 35-inch waist; five and a half times higher for a 36- to 37-inch waist; and six times higher for a 38-inch or larger waist. The conclusion – as you allow your waist to grow, your risk for adult on-set diabetes increases.

A big midsection is rarely healthy. In general, the smaller your stomach (up to a point – anorexia isn't healthy either) the better the health of your body. Your stomach size is an indicator of your overall condition. Not only does your stomach size affect your appearance, it also affects your health.

A bigger waistline increases your risk for adult on-set diabetes.

Getting It Right

The combination of a healthy and attractive stomach is worth working for – working hard. But hard work is not the only issue. Method also matters. You can miss the midsection shaping mark entirely by going down the wrong stomach fitness path. However, if you know how to direct your waist training, you will be able to make noticeable changes in your midsection. Certain training tools work better for shaping than others. Learn the concept of sculpting and you will approach abdominals conditioning in an effective manner.

Sculpting the Stomach

Sculpting involves taking the stomach and changing its entire appearance. You are rearranging the shape of it. In this process you will be removing fat and adding some muscle tone.

The concept of sculpting is the best way to visualize the waist-changing process.

When a sculptor operates, he or she does not merely toss off the unwanted elements – the sculptor also spends a lot of time on shaping the remaining elements. Fat is removed and muscle is shaped. Rather than countless sets of mindless situps, focus both your mind and your body on the entire process of physical change.

Radical Change

Two main components will transform the appearance of the stomach. First, you must make the midsection more slender. This primarily involves decreasing the fat around the stomach. Secondly, shape the waist by

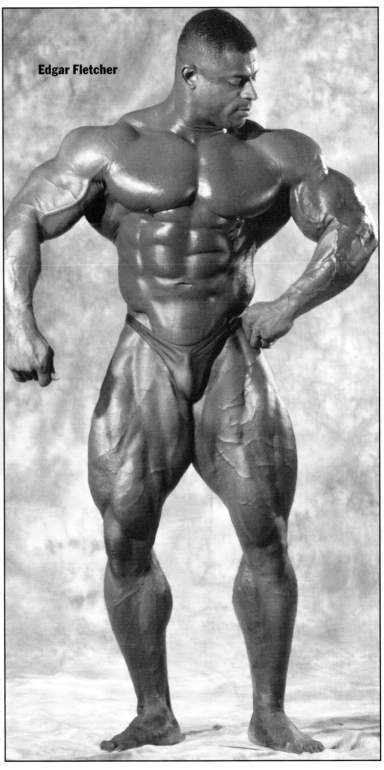

Edgar Fletcher

adding muscle. Alone, each of these areas allows for some change, but together they work magic. The combination of carving fat off the middle, along with increasing muscle tone in the same region, causes a radical new look for your waist. Mixing two elements together brings a multiplied effect.

> ## Carving fat off the middle, along with increasing the muscle tone in the stomach region, causes a radical new look for your waist.

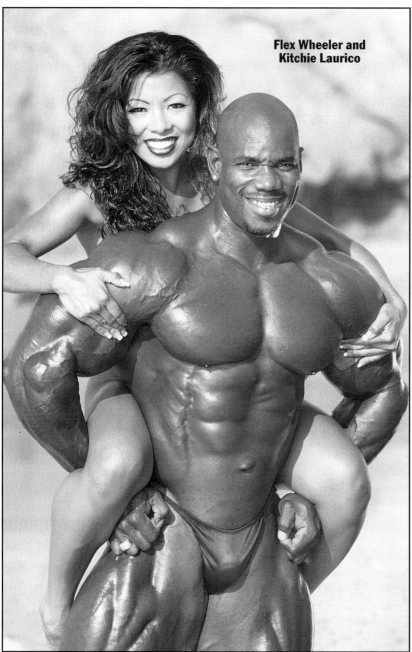

Flex Wheeler and Kitchie Laurico

Avoiding Overkill

Some people push waist training too far. Doing too much can push you toward an overtrained state. It is also a waist of time. If you can work your waist well in five minutes, then to perform 30 minutes is foolish. Overtraining can also cause problems for your physique by draining energy that is needed for other types of training. Abdominal training works best when performed with some exercise; just not too much exercise. The next chapter will present more information on training time and the importance of not going beyond what you need to get the job done.

Multi-Tasks

Waist training is multi-dimensional. There are many important aspects of the sculpting process. The first task is direct training, such as crunches. Diet also plays an important role in the shape and size of your stomach; so does aerobic training. Your metabolism will ultimately play a substantial role in the appearance of your stomach. Together, these components make up the full picture. Often people will only focus on one of the above areas, but expect their waistline to undergo huge changes, instantaneously. All four components must be worked on, for profound results to occur.

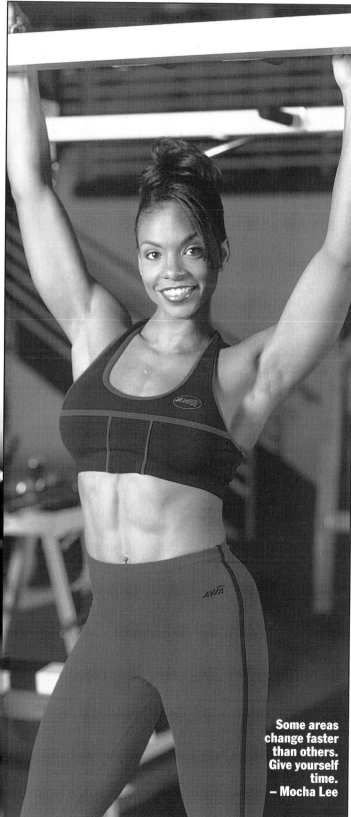

**Some areas change faster than others. Give yourself time.
– Mocha Lee**

Time

Give yourself the luxury of time when setting goals. Some areas will change quicker than others. Often the muscle tone comes in fairly quickly, but the fat takes longer to drop. Don't panic if you do not see sudden changes. Changes may come slower than what you originally anticipated. Don't give up. Stick with your training.

Lifetime Approach

Sculpting a hot stomach should be considered a lifetime approach. You can change the shape and size of your stomach in just a few months, but your primary aim should be to constantly maintain a tight and trim stomach, rather than a quick crash abdominal routine. Many people use the crash stomach workout approach. When it fails to produce the super fantastic results that they anticipated, they often stop working out altogether. It is better to use a more balanced approach, pacing your stomach training. Gradually build up to a consistent level of working out on a weekly basis. Aim at not only changing the condition of your stomach, but also at keeping it in top condition. Make it a goal to have six-pack abs for the duration of your life, rather than a once-in-a-lifetime occurrence. Look to people in the field for inspiation. Denise Austin started her own aerobics company when she got out of college. Now in her 40s, she still has a super shapely waist. It is possible to not only attain, but to maintain a hot waistline, you just need a lifetime approach.

> ## Make it a goal to not just attain, but to maintain a hot stomach.

Do you want a fantastic midsection? You can start to sculpt your own – right now.

• Make sculpting your stomach a lifetime plan, not a hit-and-get action.
• A slender stomach affects your health as well as your appearance. The trimmer the better – in both areas.
• Sculpting the stomach is much more than just making your waist smaller. It involves getting involved with the shaping of the stomach via exercise.

9

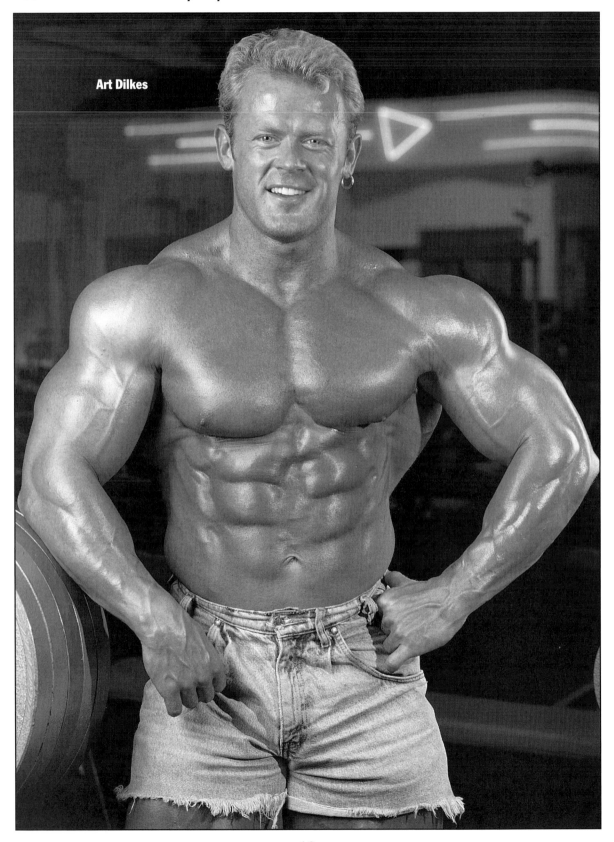

Art Dilkes

1

Spot Shaping vs. Spot Reduction

There is no such thing as spot reduction. You cannot exercise a specific area of the body and expect the fat in that area to suddenly vanish. When the body burns off fat it does so from the total body area – not just from the targeted area. Some companies promote exercise equipment that is supposed to result in spot reduction, but that is not how the body reacts. When calories are needed from fat storage, the body pulls the calories from its overall storage. Certain areas of the body may release a little more fat for fuel than other areas, but a reduction in bodyfat affects the entire body. It comes about from a change in the caloric equation (more calories spent than taken in), not from performing one specific exercise. Spot reduction is nothing more than a marketing fable.

> **Spot reduction is a marketing fable.**

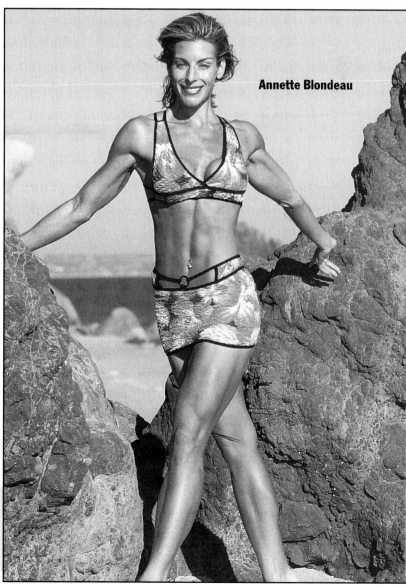

Annette Blondeau

Spot Shaping is No Fable

Spot shaping, however, is not a fable at all. Some people confuse spot shaping with spot reduction, but the two concepts are very different. Spot shaping is possible. If you perform a set of dumbell curls, do your calves respond with muscle tone? No, you see the results in your biceps. You can direct where your shaping action takes place by carefully choosing specific exercises. Arm exercises allow you to shape your arms. Leg exercises allow you to shape your muscles in the area of your legs. And stomach exercises enable you to work on the stomach region. You can spot shape any area of your body that has a major muscle group.

> ### *Spot shaping can be done wherever you have a major muscle group.*

Specific Exercises

There are a variety of exercises that can be performed for the waist region that really make the abdominals work. These exercises stimulate the stomach to increase its muscle tone. Other techniques decrease the size of your midsection (such as diet and aerobic exercise), but it is muscle conditioning that shapes the stomach. The next chapter presents 15 super hot stomach shaping exercise you can use to shape and sculpt your stomach.

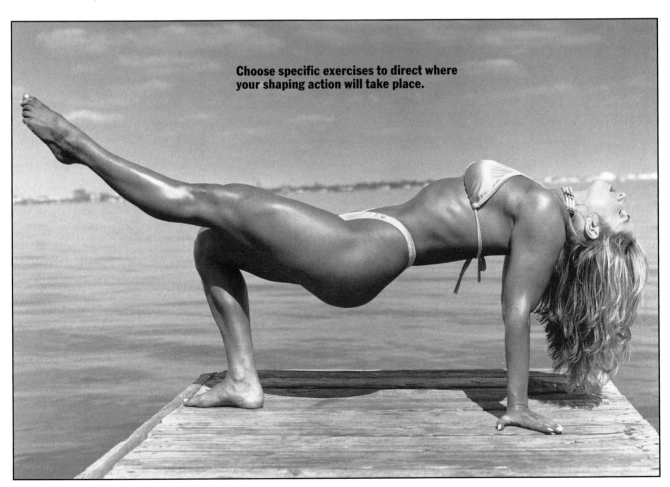

Choose specific exercises to direct where your shaping action will take place.

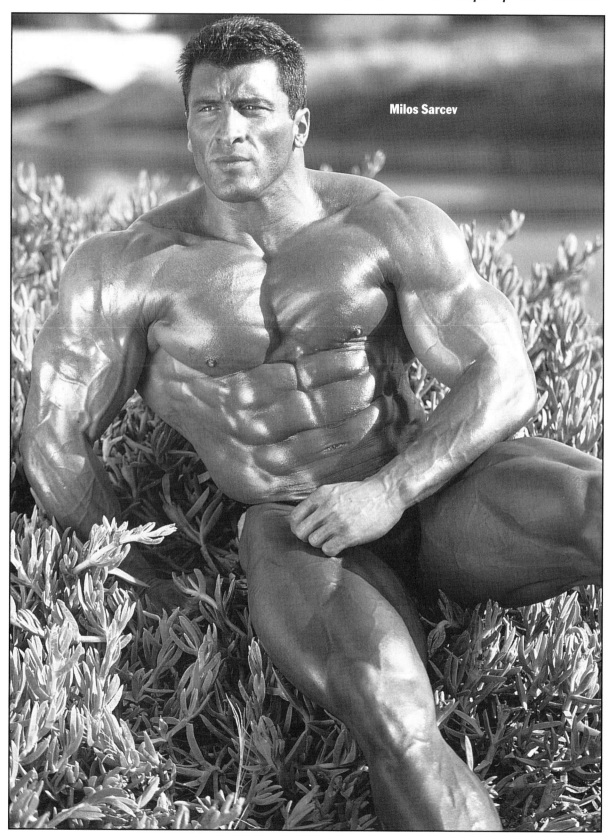

Milos Sarcev

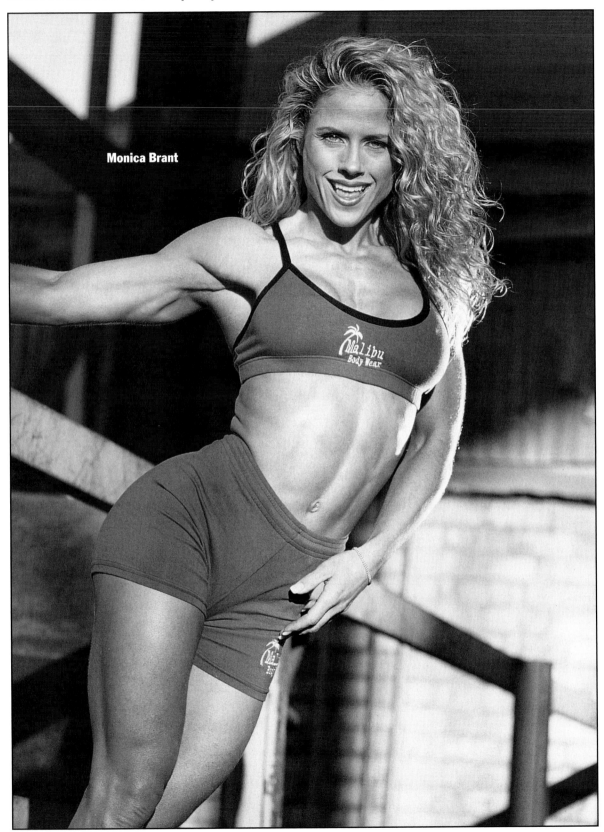

Monica Brant

15 Super Hot Ab Exercises

When it comes to working on the shape of your stomach, there is good news – you don't need to perform hundreds of exercises. Instead, a well-sculpted stomach comes from executing a few excellent exercises with consistency.

Consistency is Number One

For maximum results, consistency is a necessity. Yet many people miss this simple, but important factor. The hottest workout routine in the world is no good if you only use it a few times, then stop. You do not need to be a superstar fitness athlete to shape a sharp stomach – you just need to be consistent in both training and diet.

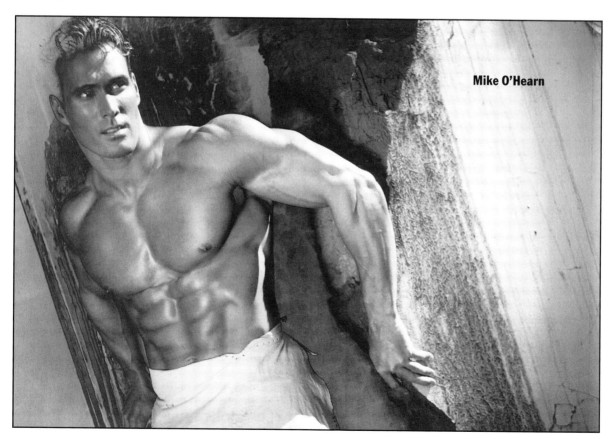

Mike O'Hearn

> ## The most important element in sculpting a super stomach is consistency.

Managed Energy

Consistency translates into realistically paced frequency. Many people get involved in a stomach shaping routine and charge forward into their training with all the energy they can muster. They perform endless waist exercises, with boundless enthusiasm – for a few weeks. Then they burn out; stop; and are not seen in the gym until the next New Year, when they repeat the process. Many people get caught in the annual New Year cycle, resulting in frustration. Hitting the physique for only a few days of hardcore training does more harm than good.

The problem is not an individual's energy level, but in how it is applied. The desire for change must be well managed. Channel your energy into a consistent, medium-paced workout routine, rather than a few high-paced crash workouts, and you will see a significant change.

As noted in the introduction, it is silly to spend more time on waist work than is necessary. Fitness guru Vince Gironda noted that the waist needs only a certain amount of work in the book *The Wild Physique*. The abdominals do not have to be worked with dozens of sets of high reps every day because they obtain the largest supply of blood in the body. Simply work the abs using, eight to 15 reps with four to five sets per exercise. The only exception are crunches, which require a higher number of repetitions.

Vince went on to note that, generally speaking, the abdominals are relatively easy to develop. He obtained top-level abdominals in just six weeks of training, and many of his students did likewise.

> ## "Work the abs using 8 to 15 reps with 4 to 5 sets per exercise."
> ## – Vince Gironda.

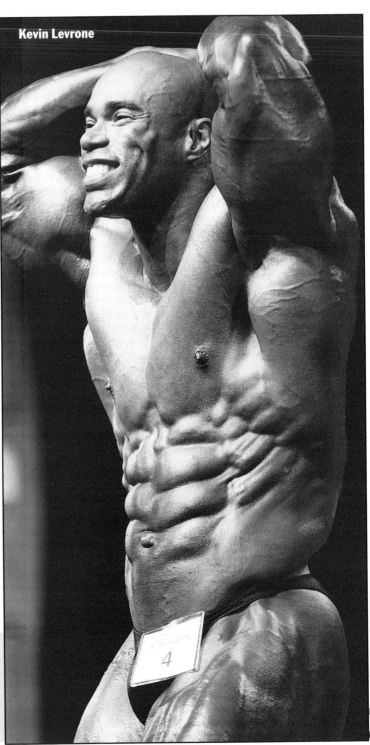

Kevin Levrone

Rotation Variation

Although you only need to perform a few exercises per waist workout, it is a good idea to have several to choose from. Not everyone responds equally to the same exercise. Variety is the best way to find out what works best for you. It also enables you to circumvent workout boredom. So alternate waist workouts! Seek out a few combinations that will work well for you. Choose from the 15 super-hot ab exercises outlined in this chapter. Also add some of your old favorites. Remember, don't use all, or even half, of these exercises in one routine. Two to three exercises per workout will work just fine.

> *A few exercises performed for 3 to 5 sets of 8 to 15 repetitions will work fantastic for tightening and shaping the stomach muscles.*

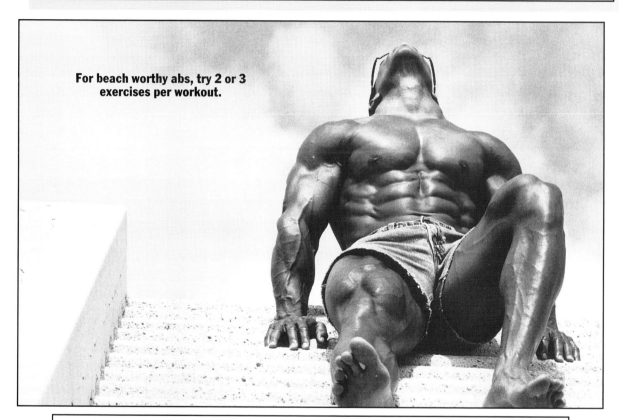

For beach worthy abs, try 2 or 3 exercises per workout.

> *If you find a particular stomach exercise combination that works well for you, stick with it.*

Frequency

How often should you train your abdominals? Three workouts a week is a good midsection training schedule. You could get away with one more, or one less, but don't extend beyond this range. Of course, if you have a limited time frame available for training, some exercise is always better than none; therefore, one workout a week is better than none. You can maintain fairly sharp abdominals on one workout per week (provided that the other elements – such as diet – are also addressed), but to make gains in this area more frequent workouts are required.

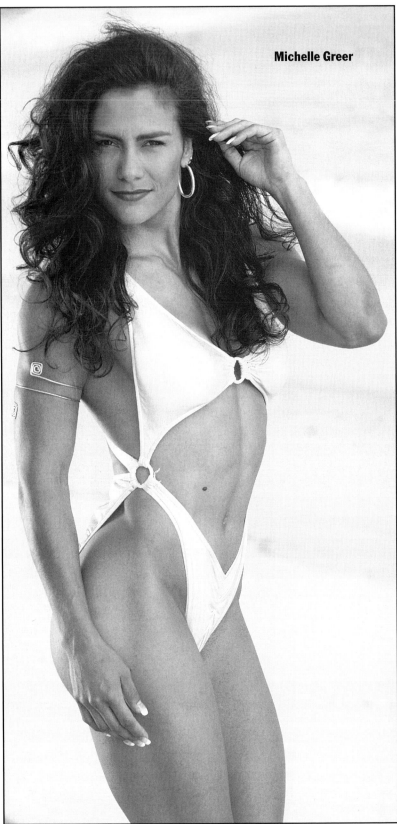

Michelle Greer

> **Don't work your waist with direct exercise every day. Getting in a workout every other day will be more than adequate for keeping your stomach sharp.**

It is not a good idea to work the waist muscles directly every day. Give your stomach at least a day of rest between workouts. The abdominals get a lot of indirect action throughout the day, and are recruited to stabilize the torso in other exercise movements. For example, when you perform biceps curls, your stomach muscles come into play in a secondary manner. A Monday/Wednesday/Friday rotation, or a Tuesday/Thursday/Saturday rotation is ideal.

The Time Element

Abdominal training does not need to take up a lot of time during the day. Performing two to three exercises for a few sets can be done fast; particularly since the rest time between sets should be fairly brief. Short training time makes it possible to get in a full waistline workout.

The Exercises

Targeted stomach exercises are needed to keep your midsection in top condition. Choose a couple of the following movements and put your waist to work.

#1 – Flat Bench Leg Raises

Some stomach exercises work the upper area of the abdominals, while others target the lower abdominals. The flat bench leg raise is a great waist exercise, that trains both upper and lower sections of the stomach. You are supporting yourself on a bench as you lift your legs. This exercise can also be performed almost on a similar apparatus that is big enough for you to recline on. The bench leg raise is a favorite of a top natural physique star who described how it is performed in *Natural Bodybuilding* magazine:

Lie on the end of a flat bench with the legs hanging off the edge. Grip the edges of the bench pad near the hips for support and lift the shoulders to pretighten the abs. Starting with the straightened legs, together and parallel to the floor. Then, contracting the abdominals, lift the legs until they are perpendicular to the floor. Lower and repeat. Keep the movement smooth.

This exercise delivers a double dose of stimulation to your mid-section, by involving the lower and upper abdominals. Use this movement consistently as part of your abdominal routine.

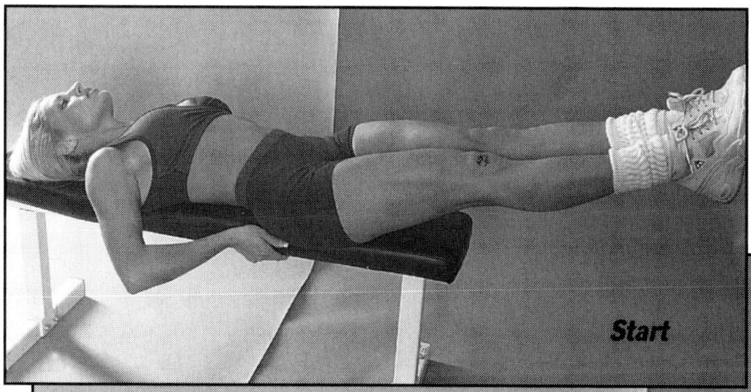

Start

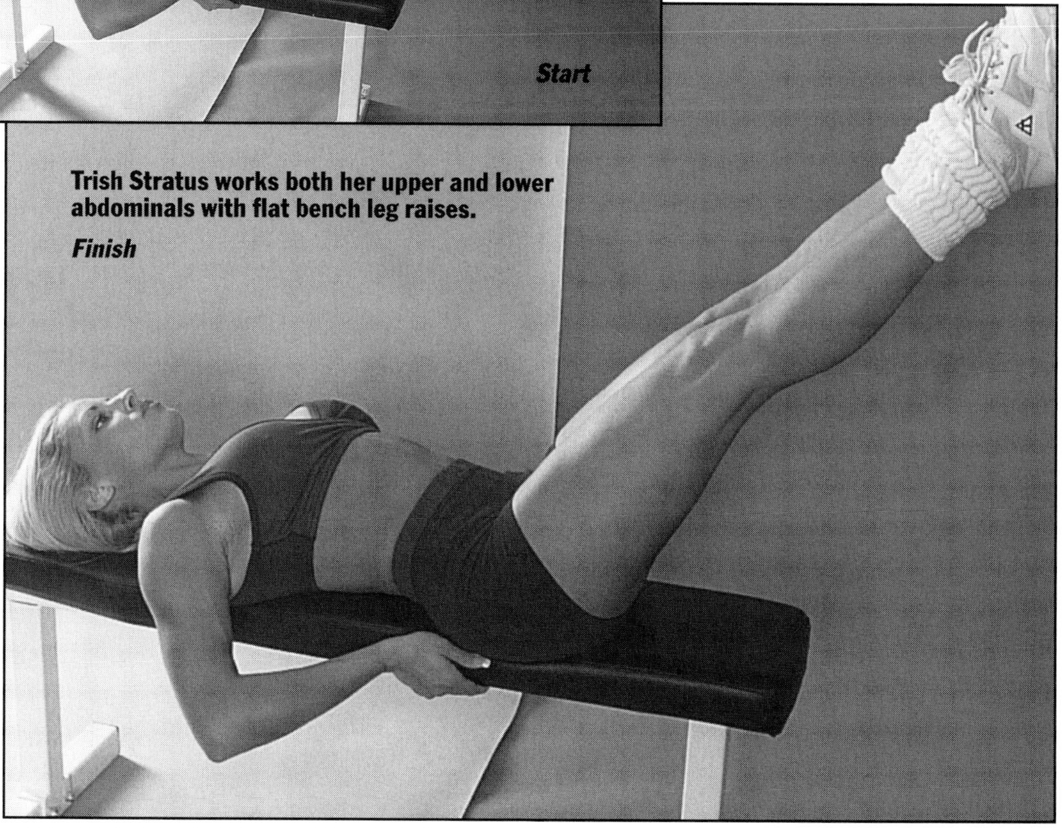

Trish Stratus works both her upper and lower abdominals with flat bench leg raises.

Finish

The flat bench leg raise should be included frequently in any stomach shaping routine because it works both the upper and lower abdominals.

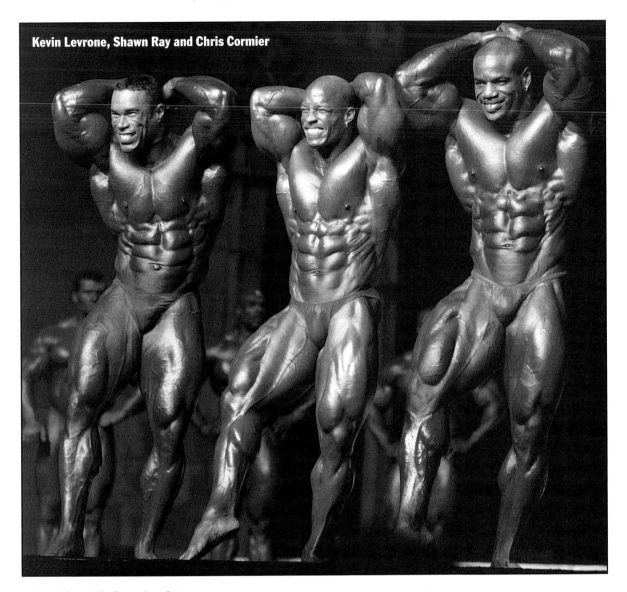

Kevin Levrone, Shawn Ray and Chris Cormier

#2 – The Abdominal Vacuum

This exercise is touted by fitness guru Vince Gironda. It is performed from a standing position, then bending forward to put your hands on a table, chair or similar object (lower is better). You can also do this exercise kneeling on the floor. If standing, bend the knees slightly, and draw your stomach muscles back in toward your spine, as much as possible, while exhaling. Hold this position for a few counts, then inhale and relax. Perform several repetitions. This exercise can also be performed by itself at other times during the day, and is a good exercise to do after getting up in the morning. It will train you to suck in your abdominals when you are posing, while reducing the size of your waistline.

> ### *The abdominal vacuum will train you to suck in your abdominals when you are posing.*

#3 – The Crunch

The abdominal move used most frequently in the fitness community is the crunch. It has replaced the situp because it is safer and more effective for isolating the abdominal muscles. The crunch provides a simple, but efficient, way to work on the stomach. It isolates the muscles you want to target. The crunch is an abbreviated torso movement. From a prone (face upward) position, with bent knees, the upper body is crunched toward the lower body. Hands are behind the head, and elbows pointed to the side. Hold at the top for two seconds, then lower the body toward the floor. But, do not let the head and hands or the feet rest on the floor.

> ### Make the crunch and bike crunch more effective by keeping your head and feet an inch off the floor in the down position.

Instead of resting at the bottom, go back into the crunch movement. Most people overlook this crucial opportunity to keep the tummy tight. It is difficult to crunch with no rest, but the pay back is worth it. The crunch is a great waist exercise that can be done almost anywhere since no apparatus is required.

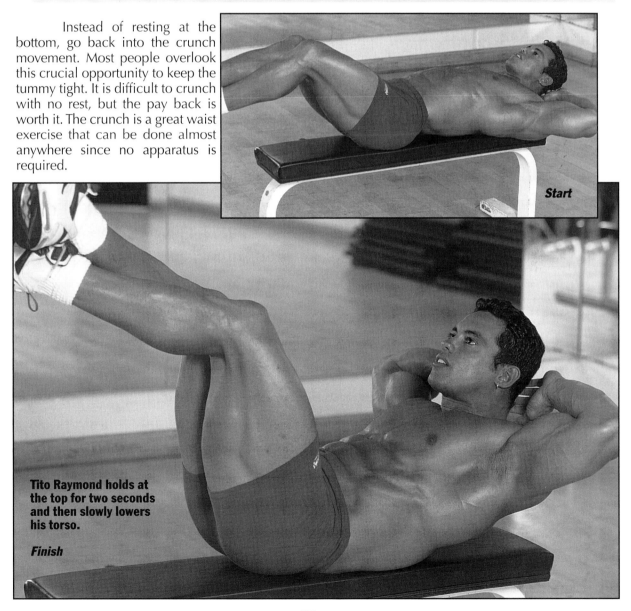

Start

Tito Raymond holds at the top for two seconds and then slowly lowers his torso.

Finish

21

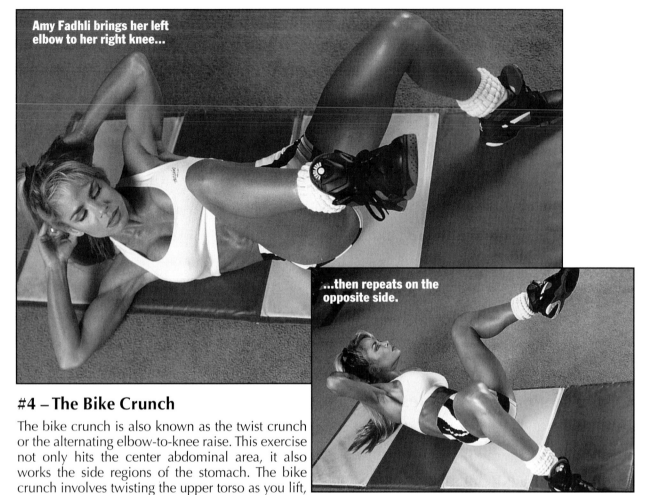

Amy Fadhli brings her left elbow to her right knee...

...then repeats on the opposite side.

#4 – The Bike Crunch

The bike crunch is also known as the twist crunch or the alternating elbow-to-knee raise. This exercise not only hits the center abdominal area, it also works the side regions of the stomach. The bike crunch involves twisting the upper torso as you lift, bringing the elbow toward the opposite knee. This bike crunch got its name because it looks somewhat like riding a bike on your back. For the best results, hold your body in the upward position for a second or two, as you contract your abdominal muscles at the top of the movement. As with the regular crunch, try not to rest at the bottom of the movement. Keep your head and feet an inch or two off of the floor.

#5 – Extended Reverse Crunches

The reverse crunch stops at floor level. The extended reverse crunch allows for a deeper stretch in the down position, working both the lower and upper abdominals. In order to do this you need to position your body on the edge of a ledge (i.e. the end of a bench). This allows you to lower your crossed legs below the parallel, increasing the workload of the lower abdominals. Like the flat bench leg raises, the extended reverse crunch is a great full abdominal exercise. Move slowly. If you cannot feel your abs working you are probably going too fast. Slow down to increase the tension.

> ***The extended reverse crunch is a great exercise for working both the upper and lower abdominals. It works best when done in slow motion.***

#6 – Elevated Crunches

The elevated crunch is a more challenging version of the basic crunch. For this crunch movement, the feet are elevated onto a low surface such as a foot stool or bench. As you raise your upper body off the floor, also pull up with your thighs. Elevating your thighs and knees will make your torso have to travel upward as well as forward to reach the knees at the top of the movement. This elevated range is tougher to achieve and will better build the stomach muscles. Do not start off with this move; use it after you have been using the regular crunch and bike crunch for at least a few weeks.

The raised range of the elevated crunch is tougher to achieve, but will really build the stomach muscles.

#7 – Elevated Partial Situps

As with the crunch, the partial situp can be done with the lower body in an elevated position. For the elevated partial situp, the feet will have to be braced. Bring your upper body up, stopping just before you reach the top. Then lower, almost all the way down. Not letting your body go all the way up or all the way down takes away the momentum factor; forcing the stomach muscles to do all of the work. Do not do this exercise until you have several weeks of basic partial situps under your belt, and are ready to move on to a more stimulating exercise.

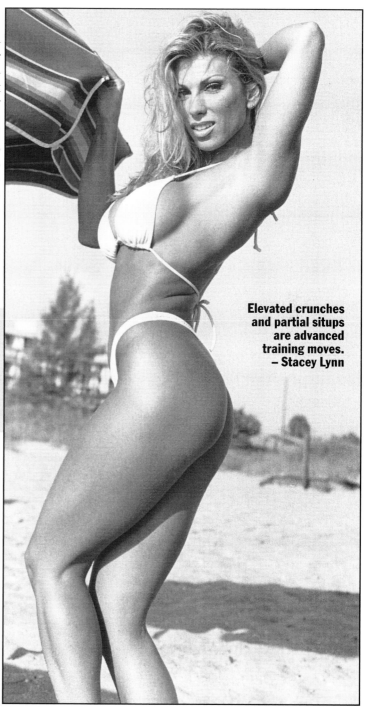

Elevated crunches and partial situps are advanced training moves.
– Stacey Lynn

By not allowing your body to come all the way up or go all the way down, momentum is unable to assist you – your muscles must work harder.

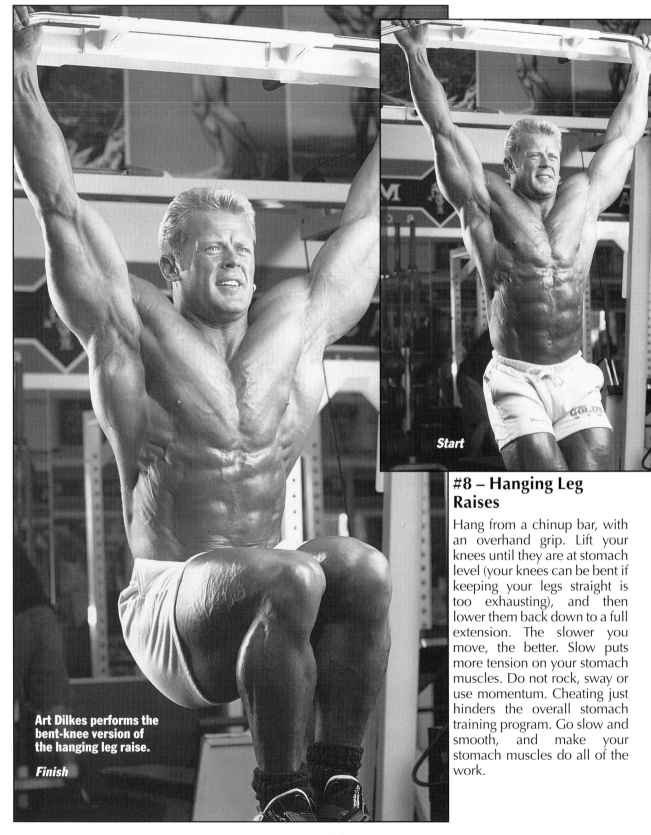

Start

Art Dilkes performs the bent-knee version of the hanging leg raise.

Finish

#8 – Hanging Leg Raises

Hang from a chinup bar, with an overhand grip. Lift your knees until they are at stomach level (your knees can be bent if keeping your legs straight is too exhausting), and then lower them back down to a full extension. The slower you move, the better. Slow puts more tension on your stomach muscles. Do not rock, sway or use momentum. Cheating just hinders the overall stomach training program. Go slow and smooth, and make your stomach muscles do all of the work.

#9 – Reverse Crunches

Another excellent midsection exercise touted by top trainer Vince Gironda. Execute from a prone position with your hands under your buttocks. Bend your knees, and cross your legs around the ankle area. Slowly pull your lower body toward your head until your knees are above your chest. Hold for a second at the top, and slowly return to starting position. Repeat.

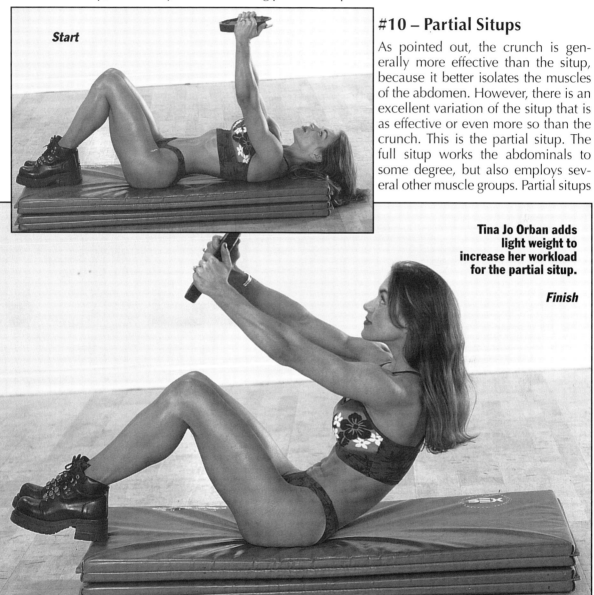

Start

#10 – Partial Situps

As pointed out, the crunch is generally more effective than the situp, because it better isolates the muscles of the abdomen. However, there is an excellent variation of the situp that is as effective or even more so than the crunch. This is the partial situp. The full situp works the abdominals to some degree, but also employs several other muscle groups. Partial situps

Tina Jo Orban adds light weight to increase her workload for the partial situp.

Finish

work the abdominals more directly. It is done by bringing the upper body only half way up, rather than the full range of the regular situp. Your feet are never braced for the partial situp (in full situps they often are). These differences place a stronger workload on the abdominal muscles. The partial situp is not as easy as regular situps, but better for tightening the tummy.

One way to add emphasis to the partial situp is to do it with a very high repetition range. It is an exception to the eight to 15 repetition range, suggested for most stomach exercises. Once you have done a couple of workouts at the eight to 15 repetition range, continue to add repetitions. Aim as high as 50 to 100 non-stop repetitions for this exercise.

#11 – V-Raises

The V-raise is done from a prone, face-up position. Raise both hands and feet, bringing them toward each other. Your middle torso remains on the floor. Slowly lower; repeat. This exercise is tough, but effective.

#12 – Wheel Rolls

Most stomach exercise gadgets are just gimmicks. You can usually get a much better waist workout without them. Many abdominal gadgets focus more on comfort than muscle conditioning. However, among the many exercise tools on the market, there are a couple that can give your abdominals a good workout. One of these is a small wheel, with a handle that runs through it. Grasp the handle on both sides and get on your knees. From this position you roll out the wheel, keeping your knees stationary. Extend out fairly far, then pull the wheel back. Use your abdominal muscles in the pulling back motion. Extend far enough that your stomach muscles are recruited, but not so far that major back muscles get involved. Experiment to find the ideal extension for your height. When you get into the right zone you will really feel your stomach working.

#13 – Elbow-to-knee Crunches

Keep your weight light for rope crunches. – Pirjo Ilkka

Finish

Start

This exercise is featured in the book *The Wild Physique*. From a prone position (face up, hands behind your head) you raise one knee and touch the elbow on the same side of the body, keeping your body flat on the floor. Your knee comes around to the side in an upward movement, instead of straight up over your torso. This side raise motion brings the obliques strongly into play. Tighten your obliques at the top of the movement (by pushing the elbow toward the knee). Do this movement on both sides.

#14 – Rope Crunches

The rope crunch is a good exercise to target the stomach muscles, but it comes with a warning – don't use too much weight. Heavy weight builds heavy muscle, and you don't want too much muscle size in your stomach region. What you want is definition.

Although heavy weight is not a good idea for the rope crunch, some weight is needed to adequately stimulate the muscles. The exercise is executed from the knees with hands holding onto the rope, then pulling downward toward the knees. If you use no weight in this exercise, no work is done, since gravity is already working at pulling your upper torso downward.). Use a light weight and do the motion slowly. Contract the abdominals as you crunch.

#15 – Knees-on-Bench Crunches

Elevate your feet on a bench; your calves rest on top of the bench. The rest of your body is prone on the floor. Place your hands behind your head and raise up until you are two-thirds of the way to the top, then lower. Move at a moderate pace – the slower you go, the more effective the exercise. This nasty exercise is a favorite of Mr. Clean, Ollie McClay, who uses it to tone his clients' out of shape midsections.

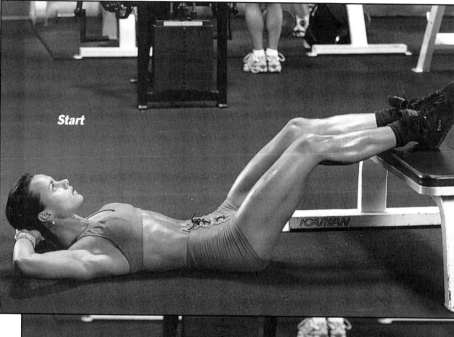

Start

Few vs. Many

Most people think that the more stomach exercises they do the better. However, the abdominal muscle region is small. It does not need hundreds of sets and repetitions to respond. It is easy to make the mistake of overtraining. Simply, focus on a few of the best exercises. The 15 super hot stomach exercises are all you need for a tight and toned tummy.

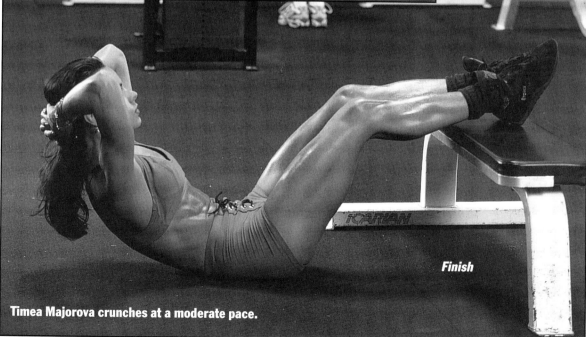

Finish

Timea Majorova crunches at a moderate pace.

> ## *Instead of using a ton of marginal midsection exercises, focus on a few of the best exercises.*

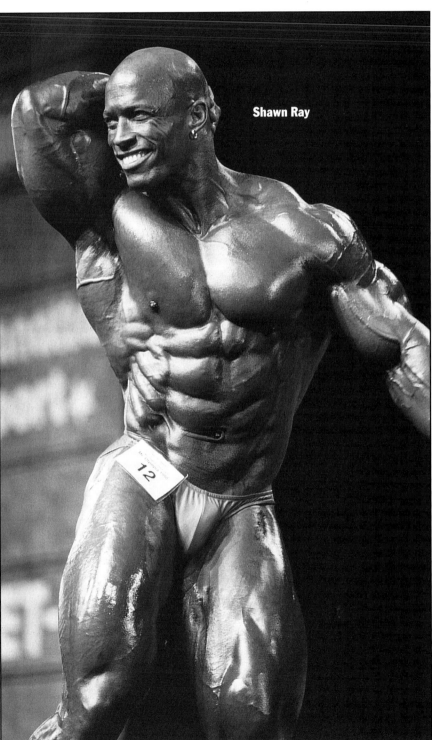

Shawn Ray

Stomach Sculpting Tips

Pick two or three of the 15 Super Hot Stomach Exercises and use them in your waist workout:

1. Flat bench leg raises
2. Abdominal vacuum
3. Crunches
4. Bike crunches
5. Extended reverse crunches
6. Elevated crunches
7. Elevated partial situps
8. Hanging leg raises
9. Reverse crunches
10. Partial situps
11. V-raises
12. Wheel rolls
13. Elbow-to-knee crunches
14. Rope crunches
15. Knees-on-bench crunches

The Ideal Weekly Waist Workout:

Do two or three of the 15 exercises, three times a week. Get in three to five sets per exercise; eight to 15 repetitions per movement (with the exception of the suggested higher repetition range for the partial situp).

When using weights go light. However, most abdominal work is best without weights.

The Busy Person's Waist Workout:

Do one to three of the 15 exercises, once or twice a week. Get in two or three sets per exercise of eight to 15 repetitions per movement.

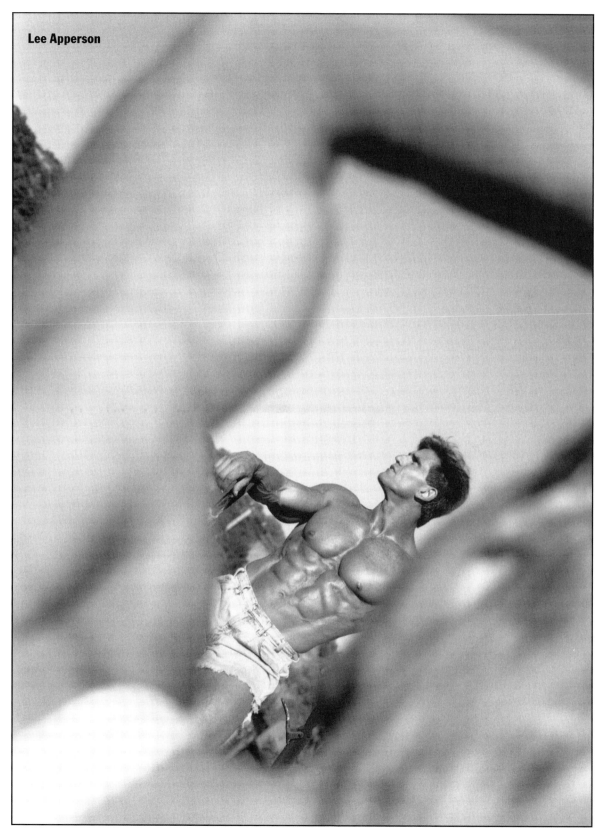

Lee Apperson

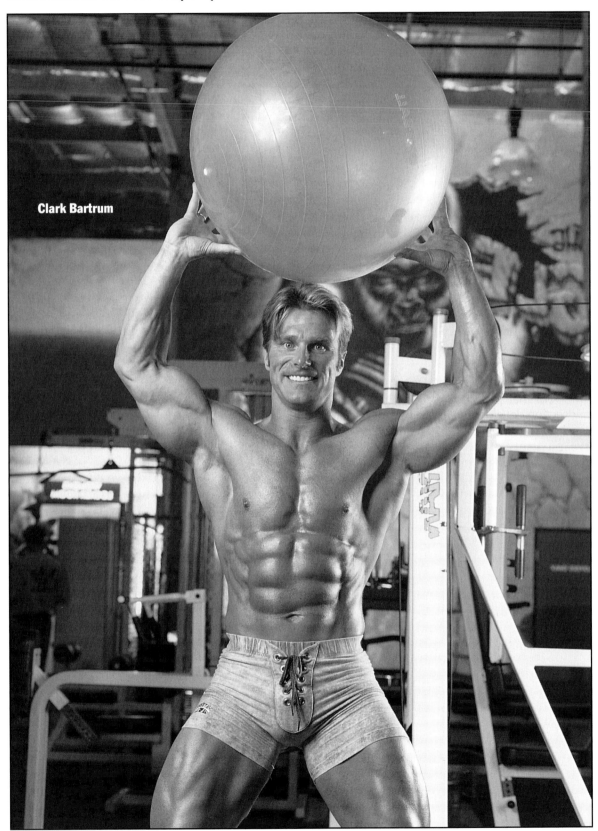

Clark Bartrum

3

Monitoring the Midsection

How do you know when you are making good progress in your stomach sculpting program? When other people remark about it? Certainly that is a good indicator, but you can follow your progress even with no one around to point out your progress. You just need some specific tools.

The Weight Scales – Pros & Cons

One tool that people commonly use to check their midsection development is the weight scale. The thinking is that if inches are coming off the midsection, then you should weigh less. The weight scales, however, present a scewed result and should not be used alone as an indicator of your progress. Scales only measure total bodyweight, not percentage of fat, nor muscle gains. The scales may lead you to a false conclusion. Here's how. A person loses some bodyfat due to exercise, a better diet and an increased metabolic rate. They lose four pounds of bodyfat. However, due to the exercise, they gain five pounds of muscle. If people rely solely on the scales, then they might become discouraged. However, losing four pounds of bodyfat, while gaining five pounds of muscle is actually fantastic progress. It means the person is substituting muscle in the place of fat – a great trade.

> **The weight scale is a marginal method for monitoring your physical progress. It does not tell you whether or not the weight loss is fat or toned muscle.**

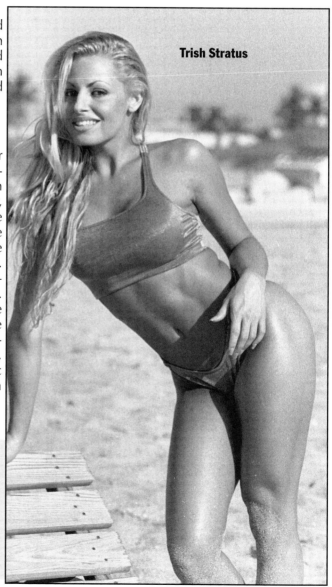

Trish Stratus

31

Another person may lose 10 pounds and think they are doing great. However, if that 10 pounds included seven pounds of muscle (due to a crash diet, etc.), two pounds of fat and one pound of water, the overall net result is that they have actually increased their percent bodyfat. As in the previous instance, the scales would give a false conclusion. Remember, the scale can help you monitor what is going on physically, but only when used in conjunction with other tools. And one of the very best tools for monitoring your middle is the tape measure.

Measuring Up

The tape measure is a great tool for checking the progress of stomach sculpting. By checking the measurement of your waist, you can get a good indication whether or not you are losing bodyfat. Although there is no such thing as spot reduction, much of the fat that you lose from overall exercise, increased metabolic rate and other factors will come from around the waist (as well as the hip/thigh/glute area). The waist is a great indicator of your fat condition. With other bodyparts it is tougher to see results from the tape measurement since areas like the arms or legs may attain an increase in size due to muscle gains, while also losing size due to burning off bodyfat. But since the waist muscle tone is mainly that which comes from bodyweight, non-weighted exercise, the size increase in the waist (due to exercise) is minimal (compared to the large size increases in areas like the legs and back). This means that loss of bodyfat readily shows up in the measurement of the waist. The smaller your waist measurement, the lower your percent of bodyfat, and the more easily your toned muscle will show through.

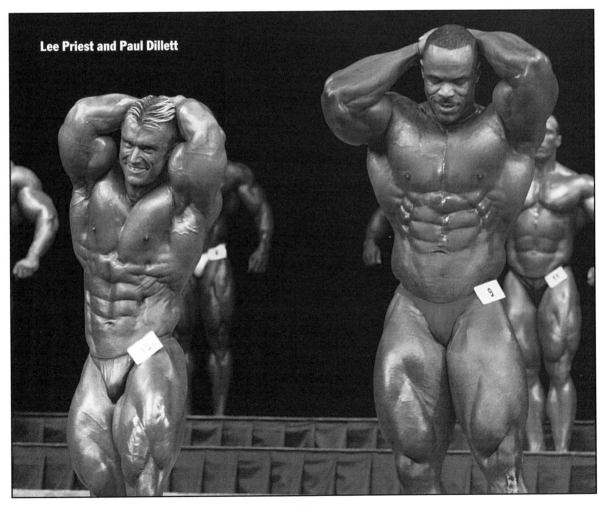
Lee Priest and Paul Dillett

> ### *The tape measure is a great indicator of the progress you're making sculpting your stomach.*

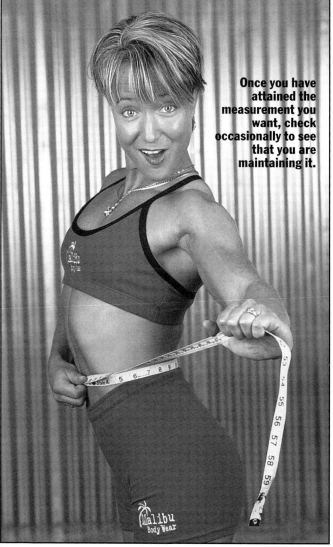

Once you have attained the measurement you want, check occasionally to see that you are maintaining it.

Since the tape measure is such a good indicator of the progress of the sculpting of your stomach, pay careful attention to what it is indicating. Measure your waist once every few weeks, and note the changes. Check how you are doing by quarter-inch increments. And don't be upset if you occasionally measure a little larger than the previous measurement – sometimes certain foods can bloat your stomach. Check again in a couple of days, for a second opinion. General progression over the period of several measurements should be toward a smaller measurement. And once you have attained the measurement that you want, check occasionally to see that you are maintaining this size.

Put more stock in the tape measure reading, as compared to the weight scale.

Caliper Check

The caliper is a great tool for checking your body-fat percentage. And you don't have to buy a super expensive edition to take advantage of this manner of monitoring your midsection. Fitness expert Covert Bailey notes that even the inexpensive models can give you a valid idea of your bodyfat percentage. By measuring the amount of bodyfat you have, with a caliper, you can tell if you are gaining or losing weight the right way – through fat loss. A caliper is much more accurate for determining fat loss. The scale tells you if you are losing weight, the caliper tells you if the weight you are losing is fat. Bailey gives his endorsement: "the calipers are very good tracking devices."

You should be able to pick up a good caliper for less than 20 dollars. Many fitness magazines frequently advertise them for sale or you may be able to obtain one at the local fitness shop or sporting goods store. Some gyms also have a fat caliper available for members to use. These calipers usually come with instructions on how to use them, but for an accurate reading take a course or get tested by a fitness professional.

Mirrors Don't Lie

The mirror provides an inexpensive, but effective way to check your fat loss and stomach shaping progression. You can see directly if you are gaining or losing ground by checking out your bare midsection in the mirror. The old proverb "the mirror doesn't lie" rings true – the mirror reflects your real condition. And since you are aiming at sculpting, what the mirror has to reveal means a lot. A fantastic midsection is not only smaller, it is also well-contoured with muscle tone. While you can look directly at the waist to observe its condition, the mirror lets you see the waist relative to the rest of your body.

> **The tape measure lets you know the size of your stomach; the mirror lets you know the shape and appearance of your stomach.**

Often other people will also notice the changes in your waist area. When you are intently working on your waist you might not notice the changes that gradually occur over time. However, others who have not seen you for awhile will notice and often let you know that your waist is shaping up well, particularly if you have made some significant changes. But overall it comes down to your opinion; which is best found in the mirror. The tape measure can let you know the size of your stomach, but the mirror also lets you know the shape of your stomach. It reveals if there is enough muscle tone, if the look is right, etc. The mirror is a good tool for assessing your progress in changing your stomach condition.

Notebook

A notebook or waist training manual is another good tool for monitoring your progress. It lets you know where you were at a specific point in time. The information that you obtain from the tape measure, weight scale, mirror and calipers can all be taken down for future reference. You can even put in your thoughts on your waist appearance, and note areas that you need to work on. A notebook is also a good place to keep track of your workouts. This in turn lets you monitor another aspect of the stomach shaping program – your workout frequency. If you keep track of all these factors in your notebook you can more precisely study your progress and make necessary adjustments.

> **A notebook provides a place to note both your workout progress and the assessment of your physique at specific intervals.**

Total Tool Assessment

Each of these various monitoring tools contribute to assessing the process of your stomach shape on a periodic basis. The use of a weight scale, tape measure, caliper, mirror and notebook add up to give you a good idea about your progress or lack of it. No single body assessment tool in itself provides enough accurate information to let you determine your precise progress. It is the total of all the tools together that sheds light on your stomach changes. Use the combination of all these observation tools to periodically check on your progress.

Debbie Kruck

Training journals like *No Pain No Gain* have everything you'll need to record your progress.
To order your own copy of *MuscleMag's No Pain No Gain* call (905) 678-2314.

Periodic – Not Constant

There is no need to go overboard and check on how you are progressing all of the time. A periodic monitoring of your progress will be sufficient. Haul out the monitoring tools once every few weeks and see how you are doing. Together these tools will give you a good indicator of how you are doing on sculpting your stomach.

Monitoring Tips

- Do not rely on any one style of monitoring your midsection.
- Use a combination of the various monitoring tools to assess your progress.
- Some of the monitoring tools used to check your progress are the weight scale, tape measure, caliper and mirror.
- Monitor your progress periodically. Don't get caught up in checking too often or not at all. Once every few weeks is a good time frame.
- Use a notebook to keep track of your progress – your waist measurement, weight and bodyfat percentage.

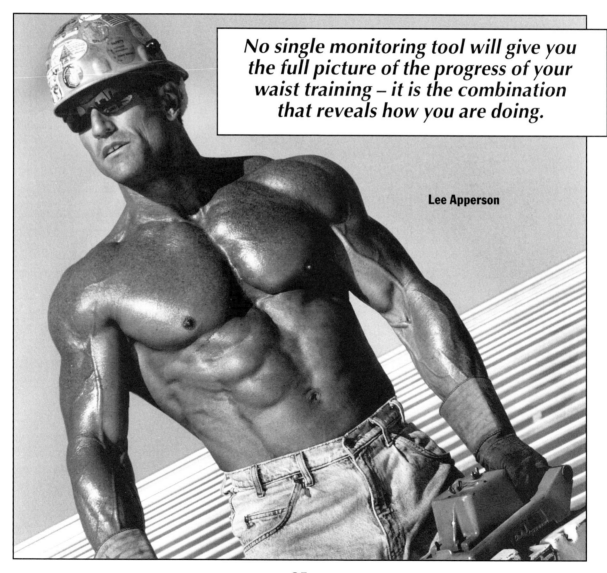

No single monitoring tool will give you the full picture of the progress of your waist training – it is the combination that reveals how you are doing.

Lee Apperson

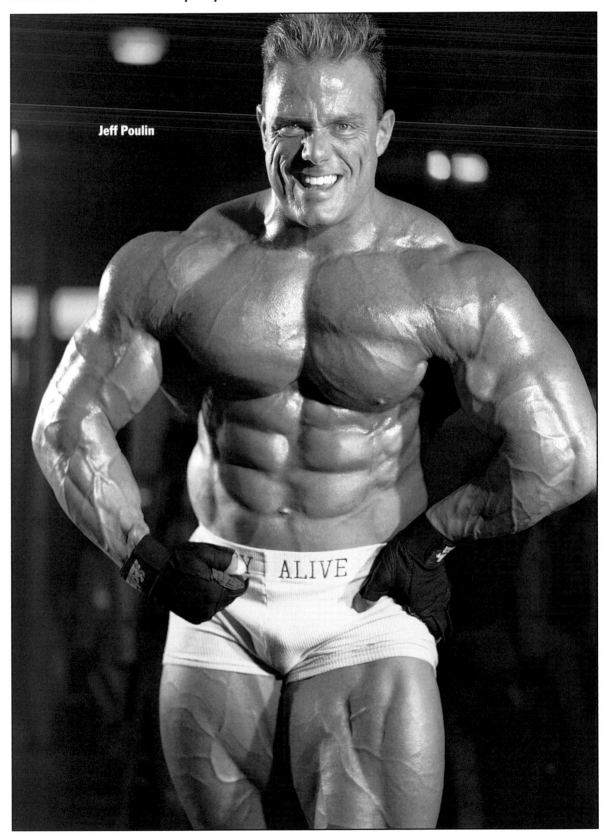

Jeff Poulin

4

Metabolic Furnace

A significant portion of sculpting the stomach consists of specific shaping exercises. However, shaping the stomach is only part of the sculpting process. Equally important is the reduction of bodyfat in this region of the physique. As noted earlier, there is no such thing as spot reduction. However, fat reduction throughout the body is very possible, and a large part of that reduction comes from the waist region.

Burning Off Bodyfat

What brings about the reduction of bodyfat? Whenever your caloric intake is less than your caloric output, your body converts fat to energy. Many things cause your caloric burning potential to elevate, and bodyfat to be burned off. The combination of these things make up your overall metabolic rate. This includes areas such as your basal metabolic rate, your resting metabolic rate, digestion, daily activities, exercise and repair from exercise, glycogen replacement and other smaller actions of the body. When your overall metabolic rate increases without a corresponding increase in caloric intake, you will start burning off bodyfat. People with higher metabolic rates tend to be thinner than those with slower metabolic rates.

Elevating Your Rate

Fortunately your metabolic rate is not set in stone. It is not static – you can change your overall metabolic rate in a positive manner. Why do you want to do so? How does this relate to sculpting your stomach? The more you increase your metabolic rate, the more

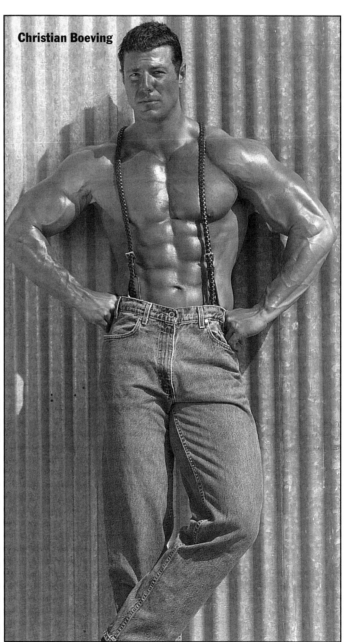

Christian Boeving

fat that you burn off during the day. And the more fat you burn off, the more slender your stomach becomes. Remember, the trimmer your waist becomes, the more noticeable the muscle tone is in your stomach. So it is to your advantage to increase your metabolism.

> **Fortunately your metabolic rate is not set in stone.**
> **You can elevate your overall metabolic rate.**

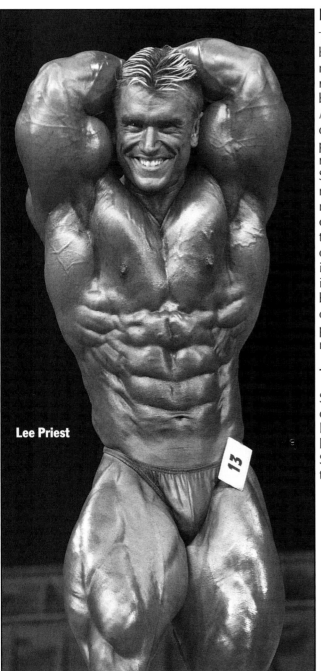

Lee Priest

Basal Metabolism

The most central part of your metabolic rate is your basal metabolic rate (a subcategory of the total metabolic rate). Your basal metabolic rate (BMR) is required for the maintenance of daily physiological body functions. Dr. Dennis Sparkman noted in *Men's Workout* (August 1997) that "most of our daily calories are burned by routine metabolic processes that are carried out whether at work or at rest." How many calories are burned? A lot. Dr. Sparkman goes on to point out "one of our main reasons for wanting to increase our BMR is that it is responsible for burning 60 to 75 percent of all the calories used by the body on a daily basis." Since the majority of calories are used for routine metabolism, increasing the BMR will have a significant impact the number of calories used each day. When it comes to the various manners in which you can burn off calories, the basal metabolism is number one. Nothing else comes close to the 60 to 75 percent caloric burn rate that your basal metabolic rate cooks off as daily fuel.

The Hype Factor

Since this rate is the main factor in burning off calories, wouldn't it be great if it could be manipulated? Fortunately, it can. Your metabolism can be hyped – elevated to a higher level. Dr. Dennis Sparkman provides some interesting information on the basal metabolic rate and its elevation:

> The BMR can be affected by a variety of things, such as room temperature, age, hormones, lean body mass and exercise. However, exercise is the disputed variable in the control of BMR. Everyone is told that exercise can elevate their metabolism, but most exercise is only sufficient at doing so for the actual time involved in performing the exercise. Prolonged bouts of low-to-moderate intensity exercise will elevate BMR for about 30 minutes . . . A recent study at Colorado State University looked at what effect exercise had on the

BMR. After weight training, the BMR of each subject was immediately measured for a continued period of two hours. During this time, the basal metabolic rate was significantly higher at every time measured during the two-hour period. The following day, the BMR's were measured again and found to be almost 10 percent higher than pre-exercise levels. Furthermore, measurements showed that much of the increased metabolism was due to the breakdown and burning of fat reserves. The conclusion of this study was that prolonged, strenuous resistance exercise can elevate the BMR for extended periods. This enhanced metabolism is due to oxidation of bodyfat.
(From *Men's Workout*, August 1997)

Exercise boosts your metabolism in a positive manner. And weightlifting not only accelerates your metabolic rate in the short term, it also has a positive long term effect.

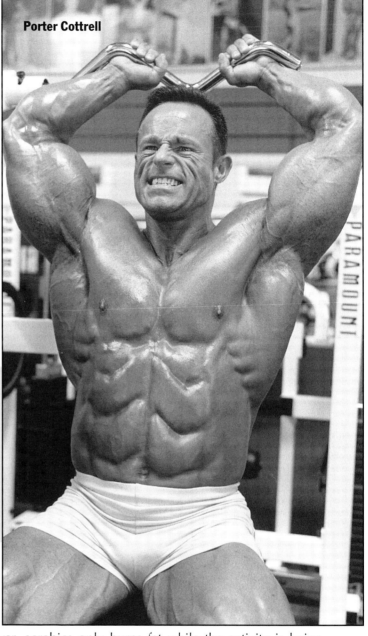

Porter Cottrell

> ## The after-burn of strenuous resistance exercise such as weight training elevates your metabolism long after the workout is over.

The exercise that most affects the BMR is strenuous resistance exercise. Dr. Sparkman makes the distinction between strength training movements and aerobic style exercise: "Any exercise that is done continuously for more than 20 minutes will burn fat. However, aerobics only burns fat while the activity is being performed. Cardio lacks an afterburn." A long aerobic workout will elevate the BMR from a few minutes to a couple of hours (depending upon the duration of the exercise session), then it returns to where it was. Resistance training elevates the metabolism for much longer – up to 24 hours.

"Depending on its duration and intensity, a good endurance (cardio/aerobic) workout will elevate your metabolism for anywhere from one to six hours. After an hour-long weight-training session, by contrast, your metabolic rate will remain higher for a full 24 hours, thanks to the huge caloric demands of rebuilding muscle tissue . . . Hoisting iron is essential in helping you avoid that spare tire."
(From *Outside* magazine, February 1997)

Strenuous resistance activity such as weight training really kicks the metabolism into high gear – and it stays there for a much longer period than that attained by aerobic exercise activity alone.

Second Rate Increase – Resting Phase

In addition to the postworkout blast that weight training provides, there is a second factor involved, to elevate your metabolism in a different manner. This affects another aspect of your overall metabolic rate – the resting rate component. When your body is not up and going, it moves back into a resting metabolic rate, a lower rate than the main daily rate. There is an interesting factor when it comes to the resting metabolic rate – strenuous activity (such as weight training) has an effect in this area also. Weight training increases your muscle mass, giving you a higher ratio of muscle to fat. This increase in turn increases your resting metabolic rate. For each pound of muscle you put on, you will burn 30 to 50 more calories every day. For instance, if you add 7 pounds of muscle, you will burn off 210 to 350 more calories every day. Lean body mass takes much more energy to sustain than fat (*Men's Health*, Nov. 1994). Muscle tissue is active even when it is resting, whereas fat tissue is comparatively inactive. The more you increase your muscle mass, the more fat you will burn on a daily basis. Since strength training is the single most productive manner in which to increase your muscle mass, it is a fantastic tool. Weight training provides yet another avenue for increasing the overall metabolic rate – through the increase in the resting metabolic rate. A *SOLOFLEX* fitness booklet points out:

> "Muscle is three times more dense than fat. To lose fat and slim down permanently you've got to build muscle. The muscle you build will increase your metabolism. In just a short time you can easily build enough muscle to burn an extra 500 to 750 calories everyday, at rest. You'd have to spend two hours or more on a treadmill to burn 750 calories!"

As this section points out, increasing your muscle tone is much more effective for burning off fat throughout the day than is something as involved as an excellent cardio/aerobic style workout. They are great for using fat for fuel for the duration of the workout, but for the "after workout burn," weight training is far superior. So by consistently using a strenuous resistance workout, such as weightlifting you increase your muscle mass, increase your metabolic rate and decrease your bodyfat levels. This adds up to a slimmer, tighter and more sculpted stomach. Remember, the weight training workout elevates the metabolism postworkout. The increase in muscle tone elevates the metabolism on a constant basis, even as the body rests. What does all of this translate into? The conclusion is that strenuous exercise, like weightlifting, will help you to shape a hot stomach via the elevated metabolism – in both the active and resting modes.

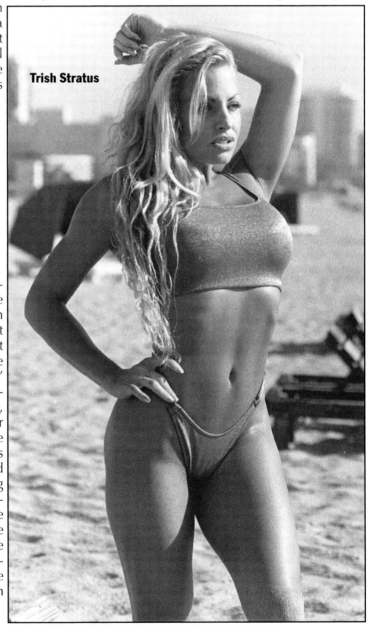

Trish Stratus

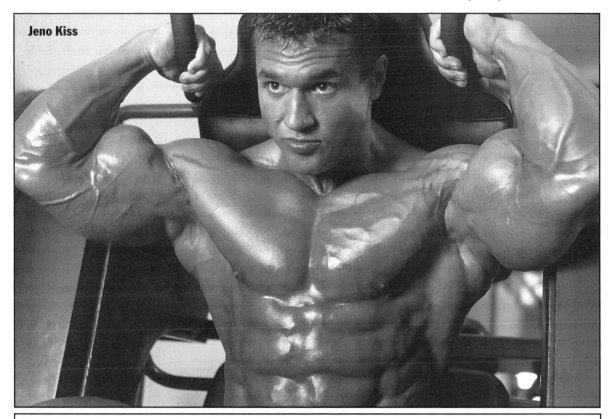

Jeno Kiss

> ## *The muscle mass that strenuous resistance exercise produces elevates your resting metabolic rate.*

The Stomach Weight Workout

To spark your metabolism to higher levels use the premier tool – weight training. Any type of lifting will help, but there is a specific type that works best. Covert Bailey writes, in *Smart Exercise:* "Get rid of the piddly dumbells. Hard muscles demand heavy iron." While light dumbells do build the muscles up somewhat, the better tools are heavier weights, since they engage the muscles more intensely. Please note that the use of heavier weights is not suggested for the abdomen region (use no weights or light weights), but for the other major muscle groups of the body which affect the metabolism when stimulated.

> ## *The metabolism is more strongly stimulated by heavier weights than by light weights.*

Compound Movements

The process of really elevating your metabolism is best fired up by weight training with compound movements. There are two basic types of strength training – compound and isolation movements. Isolation exercises, such as the dumbell curl, tend to work individual muscle groups. Compound movements work several major muscle groups at once. The clean and jerk, for example, stimulates the

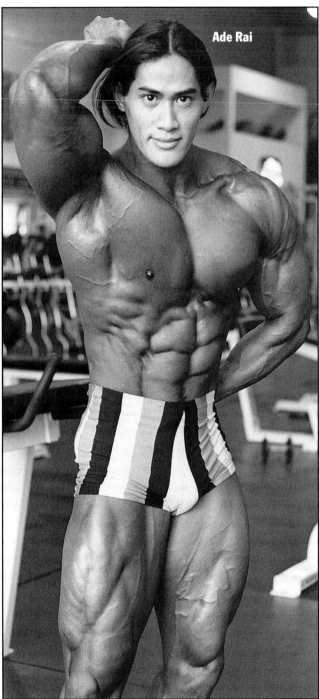

Ade Rai

biceps, triceps, legs, back and shoulders. Since the primary goal in weight training aimed at improving the metabolism is to engage large portions of muscle mass, compound exercises are your best choice.

An added benefit is that compound movements can be performed quicker since they combine the several muscle groups into one exercise. A short compound exercise program can successfully workout most of your body.

Basic Compound Workout

You need not spend hours working out to get in a good total-body workout. It is possible to effectively stimulate your metabolism with the use of just four weight training exercises. This helps you avoid spending hours on an elaborate workout program, but still enables you to reap a significant metabolic boost. Often, weight training systems that are too difficult or time intensive can discourage beginners from training. This basic workout contains four compound weight training movements. The exercises include: the clean and jerk, bench press, lat pulldown and squat. Together, they work about 95 percent of the major muscle groups of the body. The squat alone engages 65 percent of your body's total muscle mass (noted in SOLOFLEX training booklet). Since one of the main factors for elevating your metabolic rate is to develop a significant portion of your body's muscle mass, these movements are sure to help you tone up and slim down.

Clean & Jerk

This exercise engages more muscle mass than any of the other movements. The clean and jerk is done from a standing position. Do a half squat, lifting a barbell to shoulder level. Then hoist it overhead in a second motion, using your legs to get the move started. Bring the weight back to starting position. Make sure you keep the barbell close to your body throughout the exercise. Do two sets of 15 repetitions.

Bench Press

The bench press is done from a prone position on a bench. Grasp the bar with hands slightly wider than shoulder width apart. Use a weight that is challenging, but that you are still able to pump out 15 repetitions with. Lift the barbell off of the rack and slowly lower it to your upper chest area. Exhale as you return the bar to starting position. Repeat. Do two sets of 15 repetitions. If you are lifting maximal weights, it is wise to have a spotter.

Lat Pulldowns

The lat pulldown is another upper body compound exercise. If you don't have access to a lat machine, the chinup can be used as an alternative. The lat pulldown is done much like a chinup motion – in reverse. Grasp the bar with a wide-grip (your arms should make a V-formation). Contract your abdominals and lean back. Pull the bar down toward your pecs. Hold for a few seconds, then slowly release the bar; repeat. Do two sets of 15 repetitions. This is a great way to add width to your upper back.

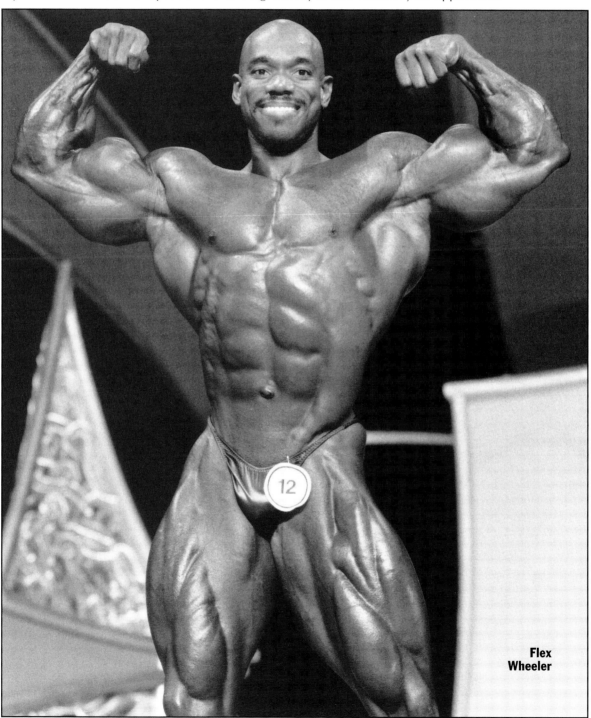

Flex Wheeler

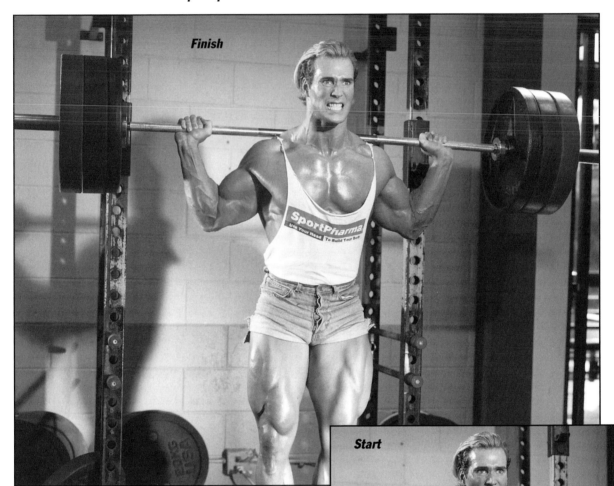

Finish

Start

Mike O'Hearn performs narrow stance squats on the Smith machine

The Squat

The squat is done by placing a barbell across your shoulder/back region and squatting down until your thighs are roughly parallel with the floor. Then return to an upright position. A shoulder-width stance is best, and it is important to keep your back neutral throughout the movement. If you keep your eyes fixed on the high end of the nearest wall, and your head up, this will assist you in keeping good posture and help prevent you from leaning forward. Spend a couple of workouts becoming familiar with the squat. Then progress to using heavy weight for two sets of 20 repetitions.

Basic Compound Workout

Exercise	Sets	Repetitions
Clean & Jerk	2	15
Bench Press	2	15
Lat Pulldowns	2	15
Squats	2	20

This simple workout will enable you to increase your metabolism, particularly if you use heavy weight. The compound exercises engage many major muscle groups, which help get your metabolism into full gear. It will stay elevated for hours postworkout.

If you want to add a little more to your workout (provided you have time) try some biceps curls, calf raises and leg curls. Do two sets of 15 repetitions of each of these exercises.

Get in a good warmup before you start the lifting session. For example, do the clean and jerk with a very light weight, followed by a very light set of bench press, then some stretching for both the upper and lower body. Then it's time to work out with intensity! (Of course for a few weeks during the initial stages, you need to get used to the exercises using light weight). Also do some stretching during and after each exercise in the workout.

It is a good idea to drink water before and during the workout, and plenty of water after the workout. Working out at an intense level uses up water stores really quickly, so replace it promptly. Drink as much as a gallon a day on the days that you train, and at least half that much on the days that you are not working out. Another good idea is to restore your muscle's glycogen stores by drinking a carb replacement drink and having some carbohydrates right after the workout. Also take some quality protein within two hours following your workout.

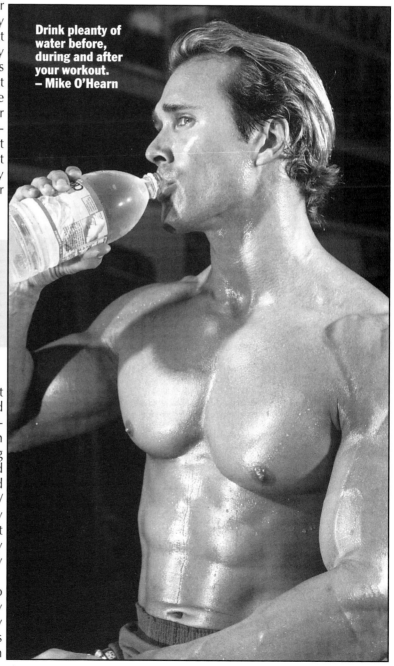

Drink pleanty of water before, during and after your workout.
– Mike O'Hearn

> ### Allow adequate time for rest and recovery (48 to 72 hours) after weight training.

Frequency

Do this compound weightlifting workout twice a week. Allow for adequate rest and recovery between each workout. This translates into 48 to 72 hours rest between workout sessions. An example of allowing adequate time for rest and recovery would be to get in a workout on a Monday and Thursday. Another good split is a Tuesday/Saturday split. Wednesday and Saturday can work as well. Configure your workout around your schedule, but allow for plenty of rest time to let your muscles fully recover from the strenuous activity.

Not everyone has the time for two workouts a week. Many people are very busy and the opportunity (shall we say luxury) of two training sessions a week is not always available. However, if you can only get in one workout per week, don't give up. You can still benefit from one intense workout per week, particularly when it consists of compound exercise activity. So aim at getting in two basic compound workouts per week, but don't be discouraged if you only manage to squeeze in one.

> ## Aim at getting in two basic compound workouts per week.

Metabolic Surge

Your metabolism is the central factor in burning off bodyfat. Increasing your metabolic rate is a good way – one of the very best ways – to get your body to burn off more fat on a consistent basis. You can give your metabolism a strong surge by using strenuous resistance exercise on a consistent basis. Strenuous resistance exercise, weightlifting in particular, is a great way to boost both your BMR and your resting metabolic rate.

By adding total body conditioning to your training schedule you really upgrade your ability to sculpt your waist. The higher metabolic rate burns off more fat, which gives you a more slender midsection.

Weightlifting does not need to take up a lot of time. A basic compound weight workout can be done in 20 to 30 minutes. Two workouts add about one hour to your week.

> ## Use weight training to give your metabolism a strong surge. One weight workout a week is far better than no weight training at all.

Take advantage of your metabolism by using the tool of weightlifting to adjust it upward. Increasing your metabolic rate will provide you with a big boost in sculpting your stomach.

• The basal metabolic rate (BMR) is responsible for burning 60 to 75 percent of the total calories burned by the body on a daily basis. Increasing your BMR will have a significant impact on the number of calories used each day.
• Prolonged strenuous resistive exercise (such as weightlifting) can elevate the BMR for extended periods. This enhanced metabolism results in increased oxidation of bodyfat.
• Additional muscle mass elevates your resting metabolic rate. You will burn 30 to 50 more calories every day, for each pound of muscle that you put on. Muscle tissue is more active than fat, even when resting.
• A basic compound weight training routine, done a couple of times a week, can enable you to elevate your metabolism.
• An increased metabolism makes the process of sculpting a sharp stomach occur more readily.

Reference

1. Hamilton, Eva May and Whitney, Eleanor. *Nutrition: Concepts and Controversies*, (New York: West Publishing Co., 1979) p.156.

Monica Brant

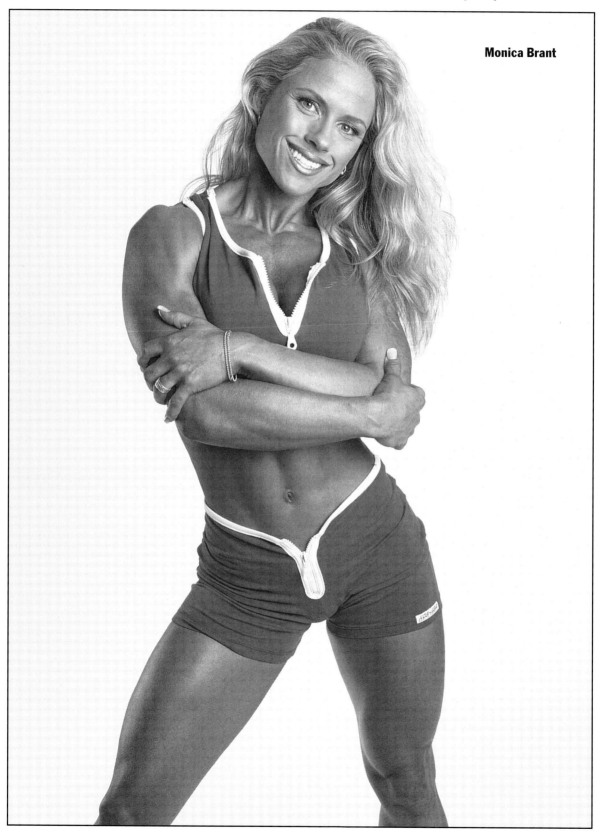

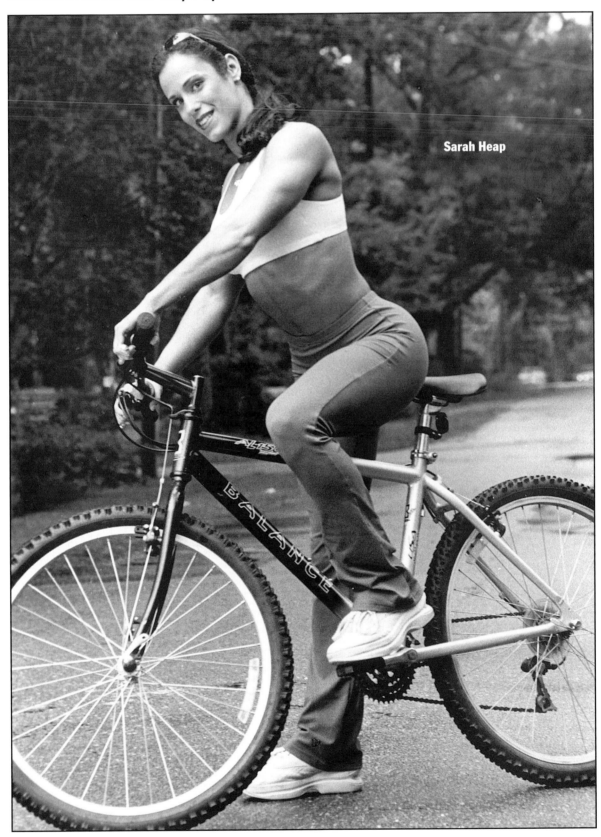

Sarah Heap

5

The Exercise and Activity Effect

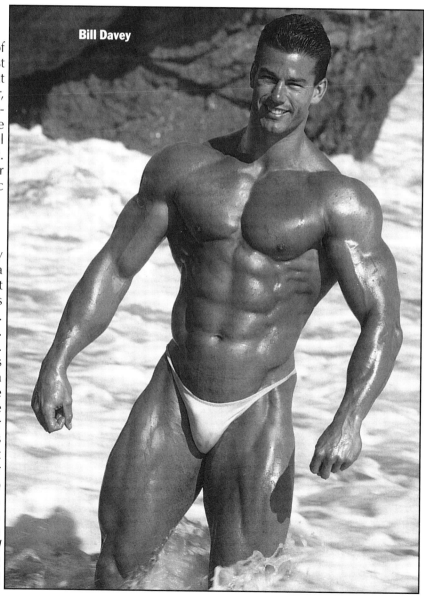

Bill Davey

Weightlifting and other types of strenuous activity really boost your metabolism and cause fat to be burned off. However, weightlifting is not the only factor you can change to cause your body to burn fat and reveal the toned muscle on your waist. Other variables include your daily activity level and aerobic conditioning.

On the Go

Most people today are fairly sedentary, which leads to a lower metabolic rate. The best way to handle this problem is simply to become more active. Make moving about a habit. First, analyze your daily habits. Are your day-to-day activities sedentary? Do you sit around a lot, or are you on the go? One person who exemplifies the active lifestyle is fitness star Denise Austin. She practices what she preaches and is a great example of how to rev up your daily activity rate. She is so active, and rarely sits down. Instead she is always standing, walking and moving about. In an interview in *Self Employed Professional*, she points out that one of her techniques for staying

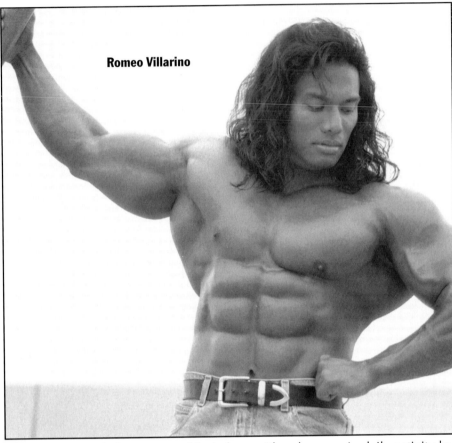

Romeo Villarino

in top shape is to move around, even when she is on phone calls. Denise's approach to the daily activities of life is dynamic. And that is a good tool for elevating your metabolism – a more on the go approach in your daily lifestyle.

Metabolic Meltdown

A sedentary lifestyle slows down your metabolism. Covert Bailey notes that the unscheduled activities of adults tend to dwindle as they get older. This gradual slowing down, the decrease in daily activity, puts the brakes on metabolism. As the metabolism drops, bodyfat starts to accumulate at an increasing rate. Most people typically do not cut back in their food intake to correspond with a decrease in activity levels. Instead, the opposite often occurs. They tend to eat more food, more frequently. The mixture of eating more food (particularly sugars and fats) along with a decrease in daily activity levels is a volatile combination that causes the metabolism to start sliding backward to a slower overall state.

The average person's increasingly sedentary level of living is different than that of the fit person. The approach of the fit person's daily habits are pointed out in *Smart Exercise*:

"Fit people are always doing something. Even reading a book is interrupted with side trips to check the stove, see who is in the driveway, and other non-essentials . . . The amount of exercise in daily activities is much greater. These are the people who play Frisbee at the beach while their average friend sits on a blanket . . . They not only do more of such activities, they perform them more strenuously."

An increased activity level not only elevates the metabolism, it is also healthy. The *American Family Physician* (1995) contained an article which presented the idea from the medical field that everyone would benefit from the accumulation of moderate physical activity, even if it occurs in short, scattered periods outside of formal exercise programs.

> ## *Fit people tend to be more active even when they are not engaging in a formal exercise activity.*

The best way to boost your metabolism through daily activity is to deliberately become more active. Instead of sitting back and letting life happen to you, go after living with more gusto. Trot up the stairs instead of taking the elevator with the crowd. Walk the five blocks to lunch instead of taking your car. Move about more frequently.

> ## *Deliberately move about more often and with more energy during the daily activities of life.*

Fidgeting & Flexing

Fidgeting – those movements that most people make when working, relaxing, etc., can also add up to an increased metabolic rate. You can add to this effect by occasionally flexing your muscles – even at work. Flexing tightens up your muscles, while burning calories. Small movements don't burn very many calories, but a lot of small movements do add up to more calories being burned.

Direct & Indirect Effect

Staying active in your daily lifestyle not only directly affects your overall metabolic rate, it also has indirect benefits. By staying active you maintain the various body functions needed for exercise and active living. It's the use it or lose it concept – the more active you are each day, the easier it is to stay active. It is a circular procession that you can use to your physical benefit, if you stay active, or it can be detrimental if you become more sedentary. Action is the variable that is incorporated into daily activities. Instead of sitting all of the time, stand more frequently. Sitting is what most people do all day long; whether in front of a desk, computer terminal or assembly line. They sit going to and from work, sit for breakfast, lunch and on breaks, sit in front of the television when they get home at night or in front of a computer while surfing the Internet. And from there the next step is to bed. If you analyze it, the body of the average person is sitting or lying down sleeping for 90 percent of the day. No wonder the body's metabolism slows down to a crawl. Instead of falling into this trap, deliberately stand more often; walk more frequently. Walking is a great way to stay active. Walk at work, and walk at home. Skip the car for short trips. Take the stairs. Many sedentary people are quick to take the elevator. Go the opposite way of the crowd, take the stairs. If you work in a multistory office, make it a deliberate habit to use the stairs frequently.

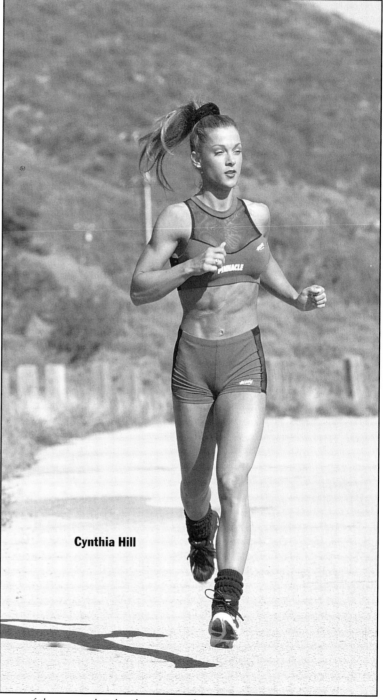

Cynthia Hill

51

Most people sit for many hours each day.

An effective technique that you can use in becoming more active is to turn the tube off. Television is probably the most alluring siren for a sedentary lifestyle. The luxury of sitting back with your feet up and slipping into a fantasy world is tempting. The only problem is that in the real world you are gaining weight. Watching the television is usually done for hours, and not alone. The viewer has plenty of snacks to accompany the shows. The combination of an inert body with high calorie snacks adds up to a flabby physique. Start getting into the habit of turning the television off – or better yet, don't turn it on in the first place. This doesn't mean you have to totally stop watching television. Just don't let it dominate your free time. Balance your day out with a variety of activities.

Moving your body around activates your metabolism. When you move your body about you engage your lean muscle mass, and when you engage your lean muscle mass, your metabolism automatically gears up in response. The sedentary state is much like a car in idle – the engine is running, but at a low level. Moving your body more frequently is like putting the car into gear and making the engine work more as the car moves. You can keep your engine out of idle and in gear by more frequent movement in your daily lifestyle.

The combination of an inert body with high calorie snacks adds up to a flabby physique.

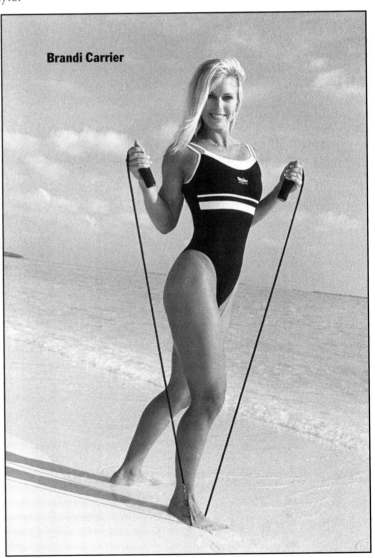

Brandi Carrier

Aerobic Exercise

Weightlifting causes a strong elevation in the metabolic level long after the exercise is over. Resistance training causes fat to be burned postworkout. The other main type of exercise – aerobic – produces less of a postworkout effect. However, an article in *Men's Workout* (May 1992) points out that a longer postworkout fat burning results as sessions increase in duration:

One of the most dramatic results came from a study by Karen Chad, Ph.D., and H.A. Wenger, Ph.D., physical education department of the University of Victoria, B.C. Chad and Wenger found cyclists used three and a half times more energy during their recovery period when they doubled their cycling time from 30 to 60 minutes. The energy required to recover from a 30-minute workout was equivalent to only three minutes of cycling. But the energy used to recover from a 60-minute workout was equivalent to 17 minutes of pedaling.

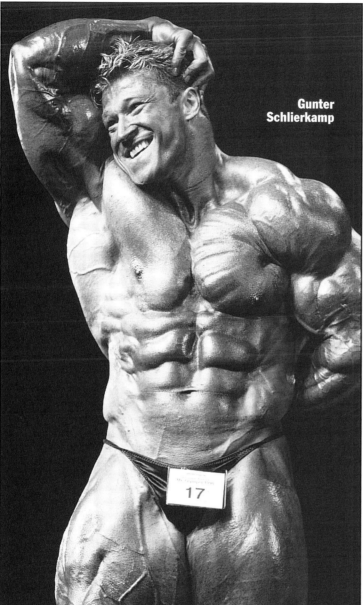

Gunter
Schlierkamp

Another factor in favor of longer workouts is that as the amount and intensity of cardiovascular exercise increases, the resting metabolism goes up (in most people). This has the delightful result that even when you're hanging loose, you're burning more calories.

Aerobic exercise is valuable in another manner. It provides an avenue for burning fat calories that weight training does not, by using bodyfat for fuel. Strenuous resistance training burns little fat for fuel during the exercise period. It uses primarily glycogen (fuel from converted carbohydrates).

During approximately the first 20 minutes of aerobic exercise, the body burns glycogen as the main fuel source, with small amounts of fat also worked into the mixture. As you continue to workout, the body switches from glycogen (as the prime fuel source) to primarily fat for fuel. The body begins to rely on released fatty acids for energy. The longer you do non-stop aerobic exercise, the more fat that is released. This means that you want to aim at doing 45 to 60 minute cardio workouts to increase the percentage of fat stores used in relation to glycogen.

As a summary, aerobic exercise is important for fat loss for several reasons. While it prompts some postworkout fat burn, it also causes fat to be burned as fuel during the workout. A longer workout converts more bodyfat to fuel. The fitter you become, through habitual aerobic workouts, the faster your body will start to use fat as fuel. Fitter people switch to the fat burning mode more quickly than those who are less fit. A person who is out of shape may take up to 30 minutes or more of non-stop cardio before the body switches to fat as a primary fuel source. Fitter individuals may start to burn fat for fuel within 10 to 12 minutes of the workout. The fit person has a strong advantage, but they have earned it. Frequent workouts develop a faster path to utilizing the fat stores.

The best way to use aerobic exercise to your benefit is frequent sessions for longer durations. Each of these factors will help you increase the amount of fat your body burns, even after the exercise is over. The factors of frequency and duration are more important for fat burning via aerobic workouts than with weight training, which relies more on high intensity to generate a postworkout burn.

Although longer aerobic workouts work well for burning off bodyfat, don't try a super long workout right away. Gradually increase the length of your cardio. Let your body slowly and smoothly become accustomed to the longer aerobic routine. How long of a time frame should you aim for? Initially try to work up to a 20 minute workout. Once you have achieved this level, slowly double that amount. Stay at this level for a few months, then start adding on time again. A 45-minute workout is a

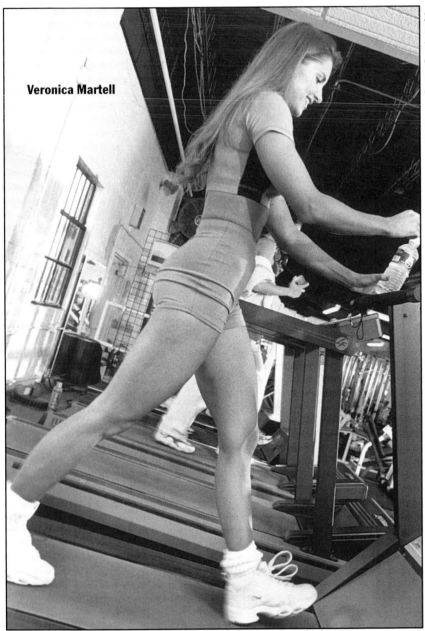

Veronica Martell

good standard to aim for once you have been working out for at least four months. An occasional workout that is even longer – 60 to 90 minutes – will help you burn off even more fat. An article in *Muscle & Fitness* (Jan. 1996) points out the importance of breaking past the 20 minute mark:

"During the first 20 minutes, the body expends about one-fifth of its glycogen stores. It takes time for the fat tissue to be stimulated, and release fatty acids to be carried to the muscle cells for energy.

Getting beyond this 20 minute mark is crucial for getting at the bodyfat stores that you want to burn off. If you just take your training up to 10 to 15 minutes per workout you will miss out on most of the fat-burning effect. So establish 20 minutes as the bare minimum for your aerobic training, and make it a goal to gradually make your aerobic workouts considerably longer than this minimal level."

Aerobic exercise burns off calories. Longer workout sessions insure that a higher percentage of these calories are coming from fat rather than glycogen. Exercise helps tip the daily calorie equation (total calories taken in vs. total calories expended) in your favor.

52 Flavors

When it comes to cardiovascular training, there are dozens of choices. A few of the top aerobic exercises are noted, but any that cause you to keep your major muscle groups moving non-stop for 20 to 90 minutes will work well.

Running

Running and jogging are great ways to get in a good aerobic workout; particularly if you initially start off easy and gradually build up your capabilities. Unfortunately, injury due to repetative stress is one area of caution. Jogging or running all of the time, particularly on a hard surface, can cause shin splints and other ailments. If you choose jogging as your cardiovascular workout, combine it with other aerobic style exercises.

Walking – Outside and Treadmill

Power walking is a fantastic way to burn off calories; so is the treadmill. Both are exercises that can be done by most anyone. Power walking and treadmill walking should both be done at a fast pace. The treadmill gets top marks as an indoor exercise. Using the treadmill for your aerobic exercise is good for habitual aerobic fitness because it allows you to work out all year long, without worrying about stormy weather or mean dogs. The treadmill gets top ratings in the health newsletter *Quest* .

"Among indoor workout equipment, the treadmill provides the most efficient way to burn calories. It's up to 40 percent more effective than other machines," reports *The Journal of the American Medical Association*. Treadmills induced higher rates of energy expenditure and aerobic demands than a stationary cycle, rowing machine, stairstepper or crosscountry skiing simulator.

A study involving 13 young, fit volunteers showed that using a treadmill burned more calories than using any of the five other popular exercise machines, as noted in *Reader's Digest* (September 1996). The treadmill is a great tool for getting slim fast, and if you have the choice of only one indoor cardio exercise, make it the treadmill.

> ### The treadmill is rated as the top indoor aerobic exercise.

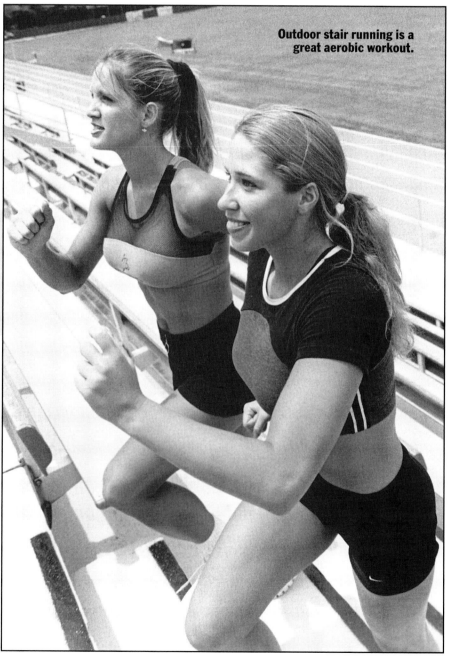

Outdoor stair running is a great aerobic workout.

Power walking will burn off the fat as well if you keep a rapid pace and swing your arms. A good rate is three and a half to five miles per hour.

Stepping Up

Any of the various stepping exercises work well as an aerobic tool. Step aerobics class, stairclimbing, or stairstepping are all good avenues for a strong aerobic workout. Start off gradually, and work your way up to a longer workout.

Variety

Running, walking and stepping are just three exercise styles of the many that are possible for you to use. You can also jump rope, swim, row, bike, crosscountry ski and the list of choices is always growing. There are many new fitness machines, each claiming a new angle. Most of them work well. So choose one, or mix a few types into your weekly routine. The essential factor is that you do the aerobic exercise for a non-stop workout. Aim at taking your workout past 20 minutes to realize it's full fat-burning potential.

> ### Aim at taking your aerobic workout past 20 minutes to maximize your full fat-burning potential.

Optimal Training Times

You can boost and increase the effectiveness of your aerobic workout by utilizing specific training times. An early morning workout is one of the best possible times to get in an aerobic workout. Champion physique star Porter Cottrell explains why:

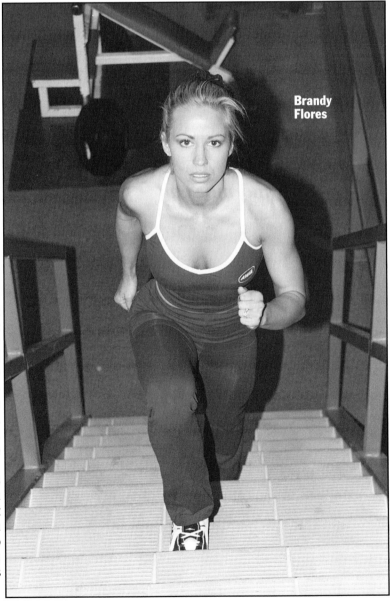

Brandy Flores

"I think one ideal time to perform your aerobics is in the morning on an empty stomach. The reason? You then have your lowest glycogen storage levels and, therefore, your body's going to use fat as a source of energy much quicker than if you'd just eaten a big plate of pasta." (*Muscle & Fitness*, October 1994)

The early morning aerobic workout allows your body to burn fat stores quicker because there is simply not much glycogen to act as a fuel source. Fat is used as fuel more quickly when you work out on an empty stomach. The early morning is one time when your stomach is really empty. Make the most of your cardio time. Do it in the morning and move into the fat-burning zone faster.

The early morning workout is not the only time that gives you extra fat-burning benefits. Another excellent time to do aerobic work is right after a weight training session. One of the top physique stars and a top-ranked trainer, Charles Glass, notes why he chooses this time to do his aerobic training:

56

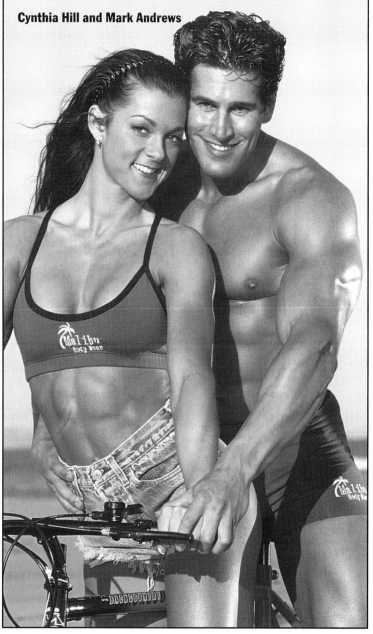

Cynthia Hill and Mark Andrews

"I have discovered that one of the most crucial elements in training is the cardio-vascular work. If you do it right, cardio really drops the bodyfat. If you walk that treadmill on an angle at a moderate rate it really burns the fat off, but keeps the muscle." Glass's cardio time ranges from 30 to 40 minutes a day, and is always conducted after weight training." At that time, your body is already prepared to burn fat," he says. "If you do your cardio before the workout it takes up to 20 minutes just to get the body into the fat-burning mode." (*Muscular Development*, March 1996).

Right after a weight training workout your body is in a fat-burning mode. Your metabolism is high from the weight training and you have used most of your glycogen stores during the strength training session. Your body burns off more fat for fuel sooner. Postweight-lifting is an excellent time to squeeze in an aerobic workout and take advantage of the fat-burning processes already at work.

> **Early morning and right after a weight workout are two optimal times for aerobic exercise.**

If you habitually do aerobic workouts you can elevate your metabolism and assist your body in burning off fat quicker. Cardiovascular exercise is a variable you can use to hype your metabolism to a higher level.

Less Fat = More Appeal

The less fat you have around your middle the more visually appealing your stomach will be. Manipulate your metabolism with more daily activity and longer aerobic exercise sessions. As you trim the fat off of your waist your stomach will become more slender, and better reveal the sculpted shape.

• Increase your daily activity level to increase your metabolic level.
• Instead of sitting all of the time, move! Stand, walk, run more frequently.
• Aerobic exercise burns fat for a primary fuel source as it is performed beyond the 20 minute mark.
• Do your aerobic exercise longer and more frequently.
• Take advantage of the optimal times for aerobic exercise – early in the morning or right after a weight training workout.

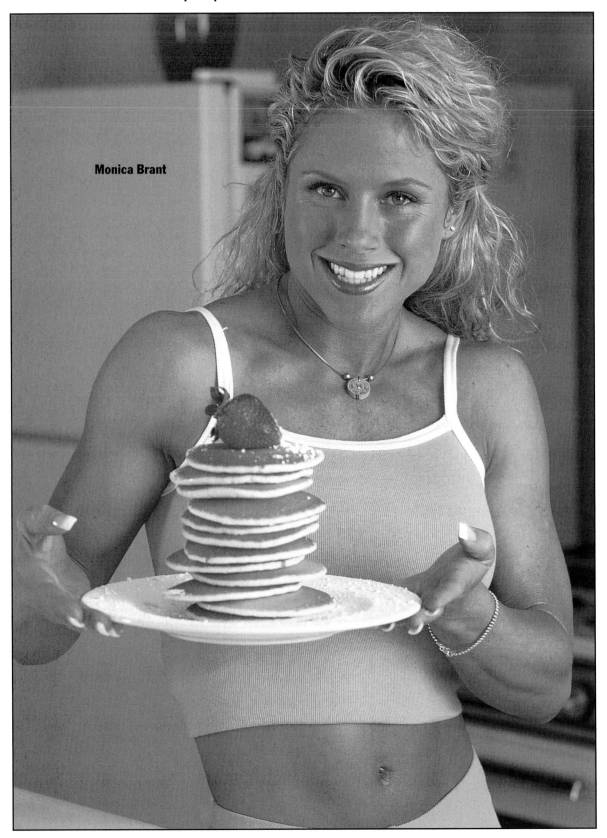

Monica Brant

6

The Thermal Factor

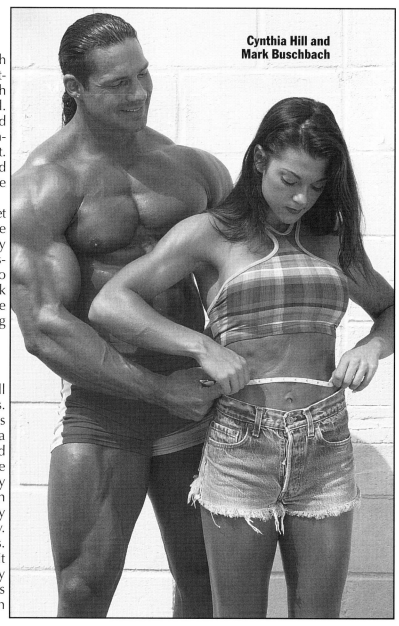

Cynthia Hill and Mark Buschbach

Whenever the topic of shaping the stomach comes up, food becomes a factor. And rightfully so, as food is digested in the stomach region and some of it is stored there as well. For some people, too much food is stored there. In order to combat this storage tendency, many people go on a crash diet. However, that is exactly what you should not do. Going on a crash diet causes more problems than benefits.

Many people use a crash diet approach. They discover they need to lose some weight, and go about it immediately and drastically. The federal trade commission has noted that almost everyone who goes on one of these crash diets gains back the weight they have lost. Crash diets are not a good option, and may end up making you gain weight in the long run.

Diet & Digestion

A noteworthy component of your overall metabolic rate is your digestive process. When you eat food your metabolism has to gear up for digestion. It has to run at a higher rate to handle the various food items it must process. Many people make the mistake of following a crash diet. They drastically cut back on food intake when trying to lose unwanted bodyweight. They may skip one or more meals during the day. Some may not eat anything for a few days. However, this is not a good idea because it tends to depress the metabolism. The body then has fewer opportunities to fire up its digestive system. Covert Bailey notes in

Smart Exercise that instead of helping people speed up their slow metabolism, these diet programs make things worse.

The Thermic Effect of Food Digestion

Missing meals makes your metabolism slow down. It has less work to do and can take time off. Normally, during the ingestion, digestion, elimination and/or storage of food, the body actually increases its metabolic rate – a natural reaction to the digestive process. This action has been labeled the thermic effect of eating. Your body has to spend calories to eat, digest, store and eliminate the food items that you give it. If you skip the opportunity to eat food, you also correspondingly skip the calorie burning thermic effect. A lot of people fall into the trap of missing meals, but in doing so they eliminate a good opportunity to fire up the body's food handling production line and the derived thermic effect.

> **Part of your overall metabolic rate is influenced by the thermic effect of eating. This is the caloric expenditure that your body puts out when you eat, digest, store and eliminate the food items that you give it.**

Obviously you don't want to be eating all of the time – that is not the solution. You take one step forward (the thermal effect) and two backward (the calories stored). What is the best way to handle this seemingly catch-22 situation? The best way to take advantage of the thermic effect of the metabolism is through reduction and substitution.

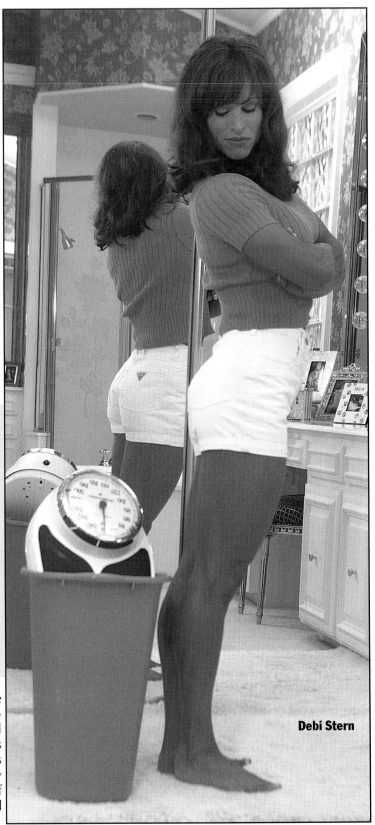

Debi Stern

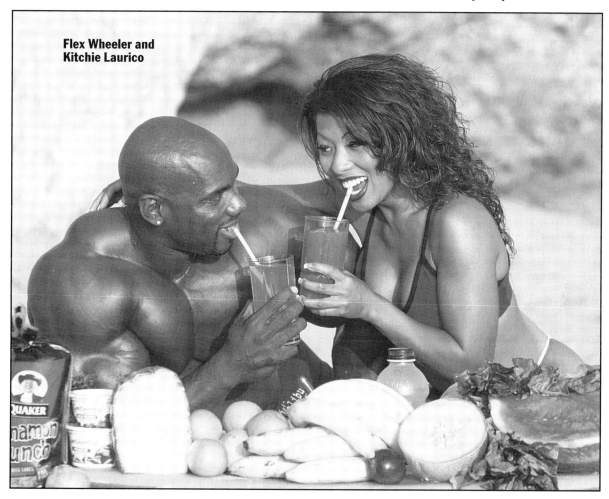

**Flex Wheeler and
Kitchie Laurico**

Reducing & Substituting

There is a great way to handle your daily diet and enhance the shape and girth of your stomach. First, avoid the average approach of crash dieting. Instead, simply reduce the amount of calories you eat during your meals and/or snacks. By lowering the amount of calories you take in you can keep the thermic effect of the metabolism frequently in play while also lowering your daily calorie total. A recent study published in the *American Journal of Clinical Nutrition* noted the benefits of eating smaller, more frequent meals (particularly for the older population). Smaller, more frequent meals fire up your metabolism.

Another way to manipulate your metabolism through the thermic effect is food substitution. Instead of eliminating your daily meals or snacks, simply substitute something low calorie in place of the high calorie food items previously part of your diet. For example, if your afternoon snack once consisted of a candy bar, substitute a banana in its place. By substituting a nutritious low calorie food item for a high calorie food item you will get rid of a lot of calories, yet still make the body work up the thermic effect to digest the banana. People frequently make the mistake of eliminating fatty and sugar foods (which should be avoided), but not adding anything in their place. The best approach is not to eliminate your time of eating, but to change the type of eating that you do during this time (snack or meal time). Focus on having nutritious and wholesome food in place of the junkfood. Choose foods rich in vitamins, minerals, fiber; but with little fat or sugar. Instead of having a candy bar or doughnut for your morning snack have some low-fat popcorn or a rice cake in its place. Instead of having a pack of cookies, choose an apple and half a bagel. When you substitute high calorie food items for low calorie

61

food items you lower your caloric intake, but still keep the thermic food processing action alive. Not only should you replace the junk food with nutritious food, you can additionally increase your metabolism if you make high fiber, complex carbohydrate foods your choice. Dr. Neal Barnard makes the point out in his diet book *Foods That Cause You To Lose Weight*: "Plant-based meals tend to increase the metabolic rate slightly." So instead of missing out on the thermic effect, keep it going through the use of food substitution. The caloric content of the substitute high fiber food is much lower than the junk food, as well as more healthy for your physique. For example, substituting a half a bagel (containing 160 calories) for a package of junk food (containing 450 calories) will greatly reduce the caloric levels. A vegetable substitute may only have 40 calories and replace a 550 plus calorie junk food item.

The vegetable food or fruit is high in beneficial fiber, as well as nutrients, vitamins and minerals. Additionally, the bulkiness (soluble and non-soluble fiber) of the vegetable substitute can help fill your stomach and prevent hunger pangs.

A difference of 500 calories may not seem like a lot, but if this type of substitution is made just twice a day it adds up to a reduction of 7,000 calories per week and more than 28,000 calories per month. In three months you will consume 84,000 less calories.

You can effectively use the metabolic manipulation technique of reducing your meal and snack intake and substituting low calorie, nutrious, high fiber foods for junk foods, to keep the thermic action working, but still cut back on caloric intake.

Simple Steps

Use the simple steps of caloric reduction and food substitution to trim your waist and to prevent any further accumulation of unwanted bodyfat. Many people make trimming down via the diet too complicated or too extreme. Allow yourself some junkfood on occasion, but make those occasions infrequent. For your main dietary approach, lower your caloric intake and include nutritious foods that are high in fiber. The better your diet, the easier time you will have forming the perfectly sculpted stomach.

Brad Baker

> ***Dieting does not have to be complicated or extreme to be successful. Use the basic steps of calorie substitution and reduction rather than elimination, to keep the thermal effect frequently in play.***

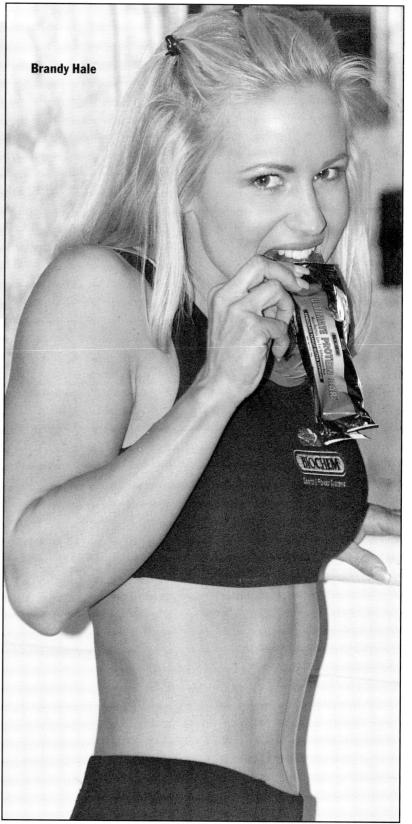

Brandy Hale

- Avoid extreme crash diets that drastically cut out food.
- You body has a thermal effect when it digests food. Use this factor in your favor by eating frequent, but small, meals.
- Instead of eliminating meals, reduce your calorie intake and substitute low-calorie, high fiber nutritious foods in place of junk food.
- Occasionally allow yourself some junk food.

Sculpting the ultimate stomach comes from the perfect mixture of training elements, diet and lifestyle. No single factor will bring either the size or shape of your abdomen into an ultimate sculpted condition. It takes attention to each of the aforementioned areas to realize the ultimate potential of your midsection. The first step is have the desire. The second is knowledge, and the third is action. Now is the time for you to enter the action stage. As you venture down the path to awesome abdominals, you will start to see a middle that is not only smaller, but also shaped better. Stick with it and you will soon achieve a waistline in ultimate condition – the perfectly sculpted stomach.

Contributing Photographers

Jim Amentler, Alex Ardenti, Reg Bradford, John A. Butler, Skip Faulkner, Irvin Gelb, Robert Kennedy, Mitsuru Okabe, David Paul, Rick Schaff, Rob Sims